THE BELLY BIBLE

The Pod Method- Doctor Endorsed

J. Podlaski

1

In Loving Memory of
Jesus & Julia, Grandmother
and Grandfather, My Daddy,
Grandma Alice, Sebastiana,

3

ACKNOWLEDGEMENTS

To my sweet dear husband Len, for it is with his devotion and love that this book was conceived, and who has filled me with more love than I have ever known…...
My angels whose squishy hugs with giggles of delight make my heart smile.   Seester Candy love you so much, mom, bro…..love…..
To my family we love you all…….

With deepest gratitude to:
Dr. Jerry A. Wider and
Dr. Morisa J. Marin

For believing in me and delivering my angels, "The first "Pod Babies".

Artwork: Ben Lewis   Thanks to: Jen Nelson

Visit our websites:
www.bellybible.com
www.bellylicious.com

Table of Contents

DISCLAIMER: BEFORE THE BEGINNING

The Pod Method was designed to help women gain control of the greatest and most intense experience that they will go through in their life- childbirth. It uses mental and visual stimulation as well as other various methods. It can be used in conjunction with all other childbirth methods. It is used in the convenience of your home.
 The author had no medical history, which would have complicated her pregnancies. The Pod Method is only to be used in normal, uncomplicated pregnancies. **YOU MUST** get your **Doctors** *authorization* to proceed with all steps discussed in this book. The author assumes no liability in any situation that may occur. Each pregnancy is unique; you may not be able to complete all the steps throughout yours. Seek your Doctor's advice throughout your pregnancy and report anything that you may feel worried about. The majority of pregnancies are uncomplicated, and The Pod Method will help you achieve a shorter less painful labor. Women with a history of miscarriage are advised not to use The Pod Method. If though, you still decide to use The Pod Method, discuss each step in full with your doctor and completely refrain from using any step that your doctor concludes may be harmful to you or your child. The Belly Bible is the author's journey taking it yourself means you are aware of the risks of pregnancy. Learning The Pod Method in normal, uncomplicated pregnancies will help your experience to be one of great joy. Wishing you a speedy delivery.

BELIEVE

CHAPTER ONE

TO KNOW ME IS TO BELIEVE

I will start this book by telling you about myself, and why I wrote The Pod Method.

I am 33 years old, a wife and mother of two children. I am in good health, moderately fit, and a stable family life help to keep me wonderfully busy and happy.

I had my first child when I was 31. I had been off the pill for six months when I found out I was expecting. My due date was set for July 28th. Of course I was thrilled, and then I was petrified. I knew this day would bring me my beautiful baby. What I felt powerless and petrified about was how I was going to accomplish this.

I knew I wanted to deliver naturally with no drugs. But I've seen and heard one too many stories of long and painful deliveries, that I knew deep inside of me I had to do something, so that it would not be me suffering nine months down the road. I knew there had to be a way to make my labor easier, shorter and less painful.

My God, we have been doing this for thousands of years, there had to be some method out there. Was I to wait patiently with every other mother to be? Was I to wait for the day I went into labor and be shocked with the reality that there was nothing I could do to help myself in this process? Why couldn't there be a way for me to hasten the process of childbirth? Why would I be powerless to help myself in the greatest journey I would ever take- giving life?

Much to my dismay there was nothing out there to help me. No method, no book, and trust me I read everything searching for something that would help me and ease my fears. Absolutely nothing was there that I knew I could do to help my child and myself make a peaceful, gentle transition into this world.

Now I was scared, really scared, and I knew I had to take control and Believe that I could take upon myself what science decreed impossible: a shorter, less painful labor during childbirth. In all my readings there was nothing that I could do during the nine months it takes to make and deliver my child. I was to go to my doctor appointments and wait. Just wait, wait, wait, and wait some more for the due date to arrive.

How could I be useless to my baby and myself for nine of the most important months of my life? I could not believe this and refused to sit back and do nothing. I was going to have a labor that most women could only hope for. But I was going to make it a reality for myself, and yes, for you too.

This book entails everything down to the minutest detail of what I did during the nine months I was waiting for my child to be born. I have tried to put my thoughts, feelings and reasons for things I did or did not do during my pregnancy. I will tell you right now, that this is one of the most important book's you will ever read if you are a woman.

I recommend that if you are planning on having children one day, that you start adapting to this method now. The sooner you start using The Pod Method, the sooner you will ensure yourself an easier labor. You must take control and believe you can do this. One of the most important methods is your mindset. Yes, how you actually think and feel about yourself as an individual and as a woman.

It is imperative that you totally change your entire thought process of yourself. I know you are thinking what does this have to do with my labor? Why do I have to start using The Pod Method months and even years before I have even conceived? I will stress to you why. We as a whole have been brainwashed by a society who feels we have no control over anything! I mean this as a truth, yes we may think we have some control in our lives, but let me ask you, if we as women cannot even control our own pregnancies, our own bodies, how can we control anything else.

I believe we have been led to believe we have no control so that then we will not rise up and accomplish many other great things, maybe take over the world?   Please, I mean no disrespect, I know we have come a long way and there are a great many women who have done well for us all, and those for their loved ones. I am talking in a deeply simplistic theory of control. Read anywhere you want, ask anyone you want, they will tell you that you have absolutely no control over your labor, in effect your body, and most of all yourself.

Am I stirring some spark in your being to believe that what I say may be true? We have no control; we are helpless, weak, and inferior. I don't believe this, but this may be what is silently believed by all, especially secretly deep down in most women. We want to be protected and saved. We believe there is no other course but to suffer as those before us have. Or do we? No, I don't believe we do. That is why you must change your mindset.

We have subconsciously passed down from generation to generation a way of thought to how much control we have over our lives and our pregnancies. Most women were constantly reminded to how much suffering their mother had while delivering them. Then there are the stories repeated over and over again of how long and painful childbirth is. There are the rare exceptions; we should listen to these stories of effortless labors. These should not be the rare but the norm in pregnancy. We should all have easier labors and we should be raised believing this to be so. If we can take control of the one area that we are told we have no control of, imagine the possibilities.

We have been brought up in a culture that does not empower women. We are constantly being told that we are powerless in almost any situation that will occur to us in our day- to- day experiences. Since little girls, our minds are embedded with words like weak, inferior, and helpless. Yet, we are the sex that has been given the monumental task of delivering life.

Our journey should not be one of utter helplessness, but of control. From the start of conception, we watch in awe as our body changes. We watch and wait, endlessly clicking off the days. Waiting for the special day that will bring your baby into your arms. Shifting from thoughts of joy to anticipated fear of this day finally arriving and how your labor will be. Our internal fear derived from years of stories describing labor as endless hours of intense pain. Stories of being torn and shredded like chopped meat. Going through hours and sometimes days of labor. Getting almost to the point of full dilation and the process stopping and ending up with a C-section.

11

We are never given any empowerment; just watch, wait and endure the process. There is no justification in this. Why would the only thing women are genetically designed to do be so difficult? Why are we told there is nothing we can do for nine months? Why are we constantly told we are powerless? I knew I had to change years of brainwashing if I was to control this process. I wasn't going to let negative subconscious thoughts hinder the process of my labor. I knew it was these thoughts that could be so detrimental to the success of my labor. It was subconscious thought, something that so to speak I had no control of, until now.

My mind which had absorbed memories so deep and pure to my being, that it was a part of who I was and who you are. Everything I had ever heard, seen or felt was part of my being. Now I was going to abolish all that I was, so that I could redirect my whole being to believe that I could be a part of this wonderful process that was happening to me.

I knew it was so vital to believe that I could do this. I was in control. I will be honest in that I did this all mentally within, and it was instant awareness. I knew what an enormous task I had ahead of me. I was doing something that was not part of your normal routine of motherhood. I was doing quite the opposite of what we had been told to do during our pregnancy. I was also so immersed in the process of controlling my body, my mind, and my entire being that I was also evolving and changing.

Becoming aware of yourself is very enlightening. You will see that other areas of your life will start to change, as you become aware of yourself. Which is great, especially when this is the time you need to be strong and in complete control. Your life will change drastically with the arrival of your baby.

Taking control of your pregnancy and knowing what you want is your first step. I knew I was going to empower my complete being to the thought process that I was in complete control. I was going to have a natural delivery and nature would progress swiftly without any interference from my negative subconscious mind.

I truly believe that your mind is so powerful, that if you are conditioned to believe all childbirths are long, difficult, and painful you will trigger this mindset at the time of your labor and it will be so. This is such a difficult thing to delete from your mind, but you must. I know that eliminating years of what you believe to be true may seem hard. But it is really not. You must first believe that the stories you have heard of other women's labors are theirs and theirs alone.

Even, the stories from your own family history, are not yours, they are theirs. You may have even been told that the shape of your body may contribute to a long, painful, and difficult labor. This is nonsense. I was told that I had the shape of my mother's body and would have a difficult labor, but I did not.

Your body type, height or shape, have absolutely nothing to do with the outcome of your labor. I will say that some women's internal anatomy may be a decisive factor, but this is rare and should not hinder an easier labor for you to have. But, back to abolishing negative thought from your subconscious mind. If you make a conscious effort to truly believe that you will have an easy labor, you will. If you believe all the stories you have heard and think this true and that this is how all labors are no matter what, then yours will be so too.

It is that simple. Eliminate the enemy, and conquer to win. The enemy is your fear, to conquer this and believe you are in control and there is nothing to fear is to win. The first thing I did to conquer my fear was to truly believe I would have a very easy labor. I believed without one shred of doubt that I was going to take control of my body and have a very easy delivery. I told myself that all those stories I had heard were so sad because they could have been in control, but were never led to believe they could have an easy labor.

13

But, this was not going to happen to women anymore. We are going to empower ourselves and take control. Suffering and fear during labor was going to be a thing of the past. No more, will women not be in control of the greatest process and gift we as females were given. This simple act of nature to procure our race and succession of family was not to be so difficult. It was to be simple, so that we as women would not fear the thought of having more children, but to remember our labor as one of joy and ease.

Women have been giving birth for generations, and the thought that after all the years we have come no closer in obtaining an easier method for childbirth is astounding. We still in the millennium believe we have no control. It amazes me, and that is why I developed this method.

Other areas of brainwashing in our society towards women are the definitions associated with our anatomy. I know you are saying, "How?" It is these subliminal messages and thought processes that occur in our day- to- day lives that make us who we are, and what we believe.

Something as simple as a word that makes us who we are and what we wish to be is amazing. How odd that a little word can play such a huge part in the process of childbirth. How horrible that a little word we have embedded in our subconscious can make our labor long, difficult and may even cause our labor to come to a complete halt, due to fear.

All of this has come to be because of a word. Incredible. I will explain:
We are given words like, small and tight as a virgin to describe the perfect vagina. To think large loose, slack and cavernous to describe our vagina would never be uttered. When you are in labor, your subliminal thought process is to "How a baby the size of the roaster I

14

made for dinner last week going to fit out of my tiny, tight vagina?" It is no wonder that with this mindset most women's labors are long and difficult. If you associate your anatomy, as being small and tight, how are you going to release these thoughts and believe you can fit a seven or eight pound baby out?

It is a total and destructive process of words attributed to us that we accept as women. These negative word associations play a huge part in hindering our labors. Many women can actually cause their labors to come to a halt because of fear. I know it is difficult to believe that words can actually hinder your labor, but they can. We have come to believe over years of discussion with friends, and through our readings that our vagina is small and tight. This is how women wish their anatomy to be. You would never want your vagina to be huge. The thought of having a large vagina is stricken form the core of your being as something you would never want. Couldn't even think to have? Having a large vagina is considered to having a wanton lifestyle or being referred to as a "loose woman." You see how words are coming to play now?

Imagine a so –called "loose woman" having a child. Would you think they would have a difficult or easy labor? I guarantee your gut reaction is that she would shoot that baby out so fast; they would need a baseball mitt to catch it. Why would the so to speak, "loose woman" have an easy labor, but not you? Is it because you associate yourself as pure, and virginal?

Your vagina is tight; it has never been used and abused. You are the perfect woman that all men revere. If you believe this, you will not have an easy labor. You are using word associations and they are going to hinder your labor, to the detriment of your suffering.

You must not let words or what is part of a correct culture hinder the birth of your child. Do you see how word associations bring forth

15

whole other meanings and conclusions? You do not want a word to play negative subconscious mind-games with you at such a critical moment in your life. You MUST think of your vagina as loose and cavernous. It is imperative that you can do this, so that you do not subconsciously cease your labor by fear of having a too small and tight vagina. You will believe then that you will never be able to fit your baby out.

Your vagina is tight and small but it can stretch and stretch back again. Think of it as a rubber band. If you wish keep a rubber band with you to stretch every now and then so that you will believe your vagina can stretch enormously and then stretch back.

Your mind is so powerful that it can either be a positive force or a negative force. I know of women who were so fearful that their baby could not fit out, that they actually caused a halt of their labor and had to have C-sections. This is totally avoidable. You must believe you can fit your child out effortlessly. You must not believe these words associated to us, as women, as truth. Your body was formed to do amazing things. Your vagina was designed to perform an amazing feat, to emit a baby. You must believe your vagina will do this and do not let fear or negative subconscious word associations hinder the birth of your child. You have total control over every aspect of your entire pregnancy including your anatomy.

Our entire being has been brainwashed to believe we have no control of our pregnancy and labor. This is sad and unjust. We are strong; we are in control. We would not have been given the enormous task of life if we were weak and helpless. Why are we told that each stage of labor lasts at least 3 – 10 hours for each one? If we have been told we are going to spend at least 20 hours in labor, why would we believe we our labor could progress faster?

The mind is very powerful. I believe in all the stages of labor, I just believe they occur a lot faster. Everything you read and are told, you must believe that you will do it, but your way. You will take control and have an easier delivery. You must believe this.

Read all you want for your technical details involved with your pregnancy. I am not a doctor, so I can't supply you with that area of your pregnancy. I will give you the basics of what to expect and give you all the knowledge to empower yourself to have an easier delivery. My knowledge comes from years of reading and gathering as much information as I could from mothers and obstetricians.

I will also tell you of different elements that were instrumental in intensifying my negative subconscious thoughts. I empowered myself with knowledge and fact from years of brainwashing and abolished what would hinder, and held onto what would make me stronger.

A story that helped make me stronger and believe is one I think we all remember. We have all heard the stories of women working in the fields; squatting, the baby dropping effortlessly and then slung over their mother's backs. The women then without pause would continue their work in the fields. What word's come to mind when you think of this? Do the word's barbaric, strength and strong willed come to mind? Now, think of yourself and your pregnancy, what words come to mind. I guarantee it is totally opposite of how you described the women in the fields. Why would you completely believe that to have a fast labor you must be barbaric? Yet this is exactly the kind of brainwashing that is instilled in our society.

When you think of a woman of culture having a bay, what images come to mind? Doctors, clean sheets, walking up and down the hallways for hours, and screams of agony. Why would you believe that the women in the fields are capable of a rapid, easy labor but not you?

It is exactly this negative imagery that you are going to abolish from your thoughts. Once you start this process of empowerment you must continue it throughout your life. No woman should ever be controlled by a society bent on keeping a woman powerless. We alone have the power to give life and we alone can control this process.

It was because of this negative belief system instilled in our gender that The Pod Method was developed. It was designed to bring subconscious grounding of our being to a subconscious elevation of truth. It is only with truth and knowledge that we as women can empower ourselves and take control of our lives, and within our lives the control that being a woman brings to all aspects of our lives, including pregnancy and motherhood.

I was going to be in complete control of the process of my pregnancy. I was going to put out of my subconscious and conscious mind all the horror stories I had heard on childbirth that might impede the birth of my child. I was going to delve deep within my being to believe I could will my labor to happen rapidly. I was going to talk to my baby and ask for its help in making its journey out as fast as he safely could. I was going to visually stimulate my mind to also help empower me in the process of childbirth. It is so imperative that I not let subconscious thought hinder the emergence of my baby.

I was going to BELIEVE.

CHAPTER TWO

KNOWLEDGE IS STRENGTH

I have given you some thought on what it takes to adapt to The Pod Method. Now, I will tell some other areas of your pregnancy that I, and about 90% of all pregnant women do and you should do, too. I will also give you general information about what you will be going through during your nine months and then we will get back to The Pod Method.

I did what every mom to be does; I went out and bought every book on pregnancy I could find. Your basics, What to Expect When You Are Expecting, The Pregnancy Book for Today's Woman, and The Girlfriends Guide To Pregnancy were my favorites. I highly recommend reading them over and over again. I read them so many times that I practically knew them by heart. They were extremely helpful to me and will be to you. They answer any questions that you may have about your pregnancy.

19

As, I have said I am not a doctor and can only give you the basics on what to expect, during these nine months. I ask that you get these books to increase your knowledge and as your Doctor for any questions you have that are not answered sufficiently in a book.

I loved these books, but never saw anything that told me how I might have an easier labor, or help the childbirth process I was going to experience in a few months. I myself wanted to be involved in these nine months it was going to take for my child to be born. I wanted to do something other than watch my belly grow and wait for the day to finally arrive with me at a total loss of control of this wonderful experience. The Pod Method will show you what to do to take control of the greatest journey you will ever have-childbirth.

Another way I prepared myself was through birthing classes. My husband and I went to Lamaze classes. I highly recommend going to some sort of child birthing class. It will help you in your quest for knowledge and is invaluable to your partner who may not have read all your books cover to cover. The more your partner knows what you are going through and what to expect, the more they can help you. My classes helped the bond between us grow because he was given knowledge to feel a part of this glorious miracle that you are actually experiencing.

There are many different systems you can use, Lamaze being the most popular. I will tell you briefly about these other methods and what their techniques are.

LAMAZE: French physician Fernand Lamaze developed this method. It uses controlled breathing exercises that you use during your contractions on the onset of labor. Your partner helps you with your breathing by counting and helping you to relax and focus on your contractions. This method also uses a focal point that you can choose in your delivery room to help you block the pain you are enduring. Since this method uses a partner to help you cope better with your labor it is widely popular in the United States. Having someone with you does help immensely. Focusing on your breathing helps to alleviate the pain as is stated by Dr. Lamaze. I do hope that you will go to a Lamaze class. The instructors are so understanding and filled with knowledge, you will not be disappointed that you went, and neither will your partner.

GRANTLY DICK-READ METHOD- This English physician originated the method that fear will lead to a difficult labor. He observed that women who were calm had much easier deliveries. He stressed the "fear-tension-pain" theory, in that if you are without fear you will then in fact experience much less pain and have an easier labor. He also believed in breathing exercises and relaxation exercises. This method is popular with women in Canada and Britain.

BRADLEY METHOD- This method was developed by American physician Robert Bradley. His method continues on the system of Dr. Grantly Dick-Read. Dr. Bradley builds on Dr. Dick-Read's methods by stressing the importance of a coaching partner. The Bradley method completely denounces the use of the Lamaze Method, in that it strictly does not believe in the breathing technique used by Dr. Lamaze, due to the high incidence of hyperventilating among women. The Bradley method believes that with your coach's help you can achieve a level of relaxation, which will help you to achieve an easier labor. This method is less popular in the United States, but seems to me another method, which may be of great help to you at the time of your labor.

All of these methods may prove the difference between a natural childbirth, with less pain and ease, or the event of a difficult labor that may ensure a C-section, because of fear and lack of knowledge. Learn all you can in the nine months you have to wait. If you are planning to become pregnant soon, start educating yourself now.

Now I have done what you and every other women expecting will do in the quest for knowledge, as soon as you find out you are pregnant, but I did one more thing. I believed, truly believed that I could be in control. I could will my labor to happen rapidly, in effect lessening the pain I would endure. I knew there were other things I could do to increase my chances of a speedy delivery and also having a healthy baby. I believed, and you must too.

CHAPTER THREE

TRI, TRI, TRI

I will give you some brief information about your pregnancy and what to expect. Please remember I am not a Doctor and can only relate from my own experience. Please consult other sources and most importantly, your obstetrician.

You are now pregnant, YEA! This is such a wonderful time, the world seems brighter the future better. Everything seems as it should be, baby has made your world a perfect place to be.

You will visit your obstetrician as soon as you think you are pregnant, our next chapter will entail do's and don'ts to ensure a healthy baby. Your physician will confirm your pregnancy and give you a due date. Some women's cycles are not regular. You will be given an approximate due date and a later sonogram will give you a precise due date.
You will have your weight taken and urine. Some doctors may perform an internal at this time, or will schedule one for your next visit. You will have a culture taken at your internal exam to make sure everything is okay internally.

FIRST TRIMESTER- Your first month will begin with your baby enjoying floating within your fallopian tubes as it is rapidly growing. It will eventually by the third week nestle into your uterine wall and continue its amazing development.

You may experience, some nausea, it may be mild to severe. I did not have any, I only sometimes felt like I was going to be sick, but never was. It did not hinder my day –to- day schedule in any way. Keep crackers to eat, they seem to help immensely. Ask other women what they found helped. If your nausea is too much for you, try those acupressure band's for sea-sickness, they seem to work well. Try everything you can before you use any medication to curb your morning sickness.

 I am sorry, but I am a true believer in a totally pure system at this time. Your baby will be able to nurture sufficiently for the first three months off of stored nutrients in your body. If you can try to keep any food down or healthy drinks, this will probably be sufficient enough sustenance for the first three months. Please try to avoid medication for nausea. If you do feel you have no other choice, read all ingredients carefully. Try for a natural remedy, if possible. Get your physicians advice.

No one will know you are pregnant, but you and those you have told. Enjoy this time, and your clothes; they will not be worn again for about a year. You will probably be able to fit into your clothes up until the fifth month, and then you will have to buy clothes for your growing belly.

The second month your child will be a little blooming bud. The brain and eyes have started to form, and the beginnings of arms and legs are developing. At about the eighth week of pregnancy the heart will begin to beat. This will be the most exciting visit you and your partner will make to the obstetrician. Make sure you bring your partner to this visit, so that they can hear the glorious sound of your baby's heart beating.

The growing baby is inside a sac formed by a thin membrane. In time, the amniotic sac fills with fluid for the baby to safely float in. This amniotic fluid protects the baby from harm due to any bumps or pressure to the mother's abdomen. At no time during the development of your baby does your blood mix with its. This is truly amazing, and one I never knew of before. The baby is protected by the membrane, which separates the two circulations and only allows nutrients and waste products to pass through. Amazing.

Your baby at this time is only about a quarter inch long. It is beginning to show the grooves for fingers and toes on the little buds of arms and legs that are forming. The end of the second month is the last week your child will be called an embryo. Your child is now a fetus; we have come so far in such a short time. He is now about an inch long and all major organs and parts have formed for life, but your baby still needs you to thrive. Your child still cannot live on his or her own.

By the third month, your baby weighs about an ounce. Your child's intestines form outside of its body in the umbilical cord, because the abdomen is too small to contain them. They will come back in by next month. The umbilical cord is well formed and contains two arteries. One of which brings nutrients to your baby and the other, which carries waste away from the baby, to the placenta. The fetus is about three inches long.

You will be given many blood tests at this time to rule out sexually transmitted diseases, genetic diseases, and anemia. You will also be tested for diabetes, and some common immunities, like rubella. A pap test to check for cervical cancer is also performed during your first three months. None of these tests actually hurt; so don't worry about them. They are strictly, routine.

SECOND TRIMESTER- Wow, you are now starting to show, well, just a little. A tiny little belly shows the rapid development of your baby in these first few months.

At the fourth month, your uterus is now about four inches in diameter. Your baby can actually just lift its head now and has grown so much that you may even begin to feel movement. Little flurries of activity in your belly bring great joy and reassurance to the anticipating mother to be. Nails are beginning to form on the fetuses' hands and feet. And the most amazing formation will occur at this time, the sexual organs will form. You now have a boy or girl. Congratulations. Underneath the baby's gums the teeth are forming though they will not show until after your child is born. About five months old, teeth may begin to come down, though some children may even begin earlier. Hair and eyelashes begin to grow, and a fine downy hair, which covers and protects the fetus,
lanugo, grows. It usually disappears by the birth of your child. Your child is now about four ounces and five inches long.

By the fifth month you will begin to feel much more movement, or even the first feeling of activity from within. The baby is sustained within the amniotic sac; it floats freely and is very happy and peaceful listening to the heartbeat of its mother. The fetus drinks this amniotic fluid and excretes urine into it also. Don't worry, this fluid is cleansed and replaced every three hours as it is exchanged with your circulation. The first stool; meconium is just forming within your child's intestines. This month, more protection is added to your child's skin. Vernix forms to protect the fetus from the constant exposure to the amniotic fluid. Your child is now about seven inches long and weighs about 12 ounces.

It is now the sixth month, your child is strong healthy, and is completely developed. It will need a few more months to grow even

26

stronger, but your child is now to the point that if you could see it, you would know exactly how he or she will look at birth. Your child's lungs are going into the final phase of development to make ready for the fetus' entry into this world. Your child is now about nine inches long and weighs one and a half pounds.

THIRD TRIMESTER- Now you are really showing. Your belly will get even bigger in the next few weeks. I know you think it can't, but it will. Your baby is now developed and what the fetus is doing now is putting on much needed weight to survive outside of your uterus.

Do not even think of dieting now. It is most important that your child continue to get all of its nutrients at this critical time. I know it may also feel cramped, your child may be resting in a not to pleasant spot of your anatomy or your child may have its feet or head lodged by your lungs and it is difficult to breathe. You have come all this way and so far things haven't been too bad, until now. Your feet hurt, your legs are swollen, and you have to buy bigger maternity clothes. I, and millions of other women know exactly what you are feeling. But you are here, your final trimester. It won't be too much longer till you are holding your beautiful baby in your arms. Try and get some much-needed sleep. Oops, I forgot, you like to sleep on your belly. Not too much longer, now.

The seventh month is an amazing time for first time parents. Watching your child move under your belly is an awesome sight that has to be, "Seen to be believed". Your child can recognize light from dark, hear and recognize your voice, and make grasping motions with its hands. Your child is now 11 inches long and weighs about three pounds.

At the eighth month your child is completely developed and if needed could be born now and survive completely on its own. The fetus is now obtaining much- needed antibodies from you through the placenta

27

to help it fight its immunity towards infection. These antibodies will last until a few months after your child is born and then he or she will start acquiring its own. Your child is 17 inches and weighs about five pounds.

The ninth month has arrived, and you now just want your child out of your swollen belly. This time is much anticipated and can be very stressful for mom, who hopes they have everything ready and prepared for their new child. Waiting for the due date can feel like forever especially if you go past your due date. Don't worry your due date is approximate and your child can come anywhere from two weeks before to two weeks after safely. Your child should be head down by now and awaiting its entry into this world. You are now days away from smiling down upon your beautiful child.

I have brought you through the months of development of your child. I will now tell you some things to be aware of during this time.

AMNIOCENTESIS: Your doctor may recommend that you have this procedure done. It is performed during the 16th and 18th week of your pregnancy. A long hollow needle is inserted into the uterus to extract a small amount of fluid.

This procedure is only done if you are over 35, and this is to ensure that your child does not have Downs – Syndrome, which occurs at a higher rate as you age. It also ensures that your child has not inherited any genetic disorders. Your doctor can go more into detail after he or she has obtained a complete medical history of you, your husband and immediate family.

This procedure is safe. You may experience slight cramping or bleeding after this procedure is done. In very rare cases, some women may have a spontaneous miscarriage. Make sure your doctor is well qualified to perform this procedure, and that it is 100% necessary.

Some doctors perform this without anesthetic. If you feel you can endure without anesthesia, you can. If not they will apply a local, which is similar to Novocain given by a dentist. I have been told this may be just as painful as the actual needle itself, so that is why many doctors don't even use the anesthetic. I completely believe in a pure system, but it will be you experiencing this procedure and only you can make this decision.

ULTRASOUND- This is the highpoint of any doctors visit. Seeing your child. With your first ultrasound done usually in the first four months, you will not see "a baby." You will see the fetus shape, its internal structures and organs. If you're lucky, and baby cooperates you can even find out the sex of your child, by your fifth month. When you get your final ultrasound towards the end of your pregnancy, you will be able to "see" your child.

This procedure is completely painless. Except for them asking you to drink a few glasses of water before your visit, there is no discomfort. You will need a full bladder for your first ultrasound. You will not need a full bladder for your second one in the last trimester of your pregnancy.

Ultrasound uses sound waves to bounce off the baby and in effect create an image, which is very useful in determining the development of your child.
Ultrasound is used to determine your due date, by measuring the size of the fetus. It also enables the technician to check all vital organs and see that they are developing properly. Ultrasound also checks your placenta. This ensures that your placenta is properly attached to your uterus and that there is enough fluid within the sac to sustain your baby. By the end of your trimester, Ultrasound check's for a breech baby and the approximate size and weight your child will be at birth. I did not care about anything else but seeing my child's beautiful face.

FETOSCOPY- this procedure is relatively new and only used where there is a predetermined risk to the baby, genetic or otherwise. This procedure procures a higher rate of fetal loss. With three to five percent chance of a miscarriage this procedure should only be done if there is no other alternative, and your doctor has completely explained all the risks and reasons why they must do this.

Fetoscopy uses a miniaturized camera with light that is inserted in an incision through your abdomen. It is then inserted into your uterus and amniotic sac. This procedure is highly sensitive and can detect many blood and skin diseases that amniocentesis can't detect.

This procedure is done around the 16th week of pregnancy. A fiber-optic endoscope is inserted into the uterus. The placenta, fetus and amniotic fluid can be observed with this telescope. Blood samples are then taken from the umbilical cord, placenta, and sometimes a small sample is taken from the fetus itself.

Other tests that are done, is: Maternal-Serum Alpha-Fetoprotein Screening. This procedure requires a blood sample from the mother. This test can detect neural tube defects such as spina bifida (a deformity of the spinal column) or anencephaly (the insufficient formation of part or all of the brain). Low levels of alpha-fetoprotein in the mother's blood may suggest the presence of Downs Syndrome of the fetus. This test is only a screening, and if your doctor feels necessary, may then result in further testing of which may include ultrasound, genetic testing and/or amniocentesis. Be prepared to consult a specialist if needed and a second opinion.

CHRONIC VILLUS SAMPLING (CVS)- This test can be done very early in your pregnancy. If you are aware of defects that may have occurred to the embryo in its earliest of stages, your doctor may perform this procedure to confirm or rule out any defects. If defects are found it is believed that terminating the pregnancy at an early stage of pregnancy may be best for the expectant mother, health-wise and emotionally.

This test is extremely invasive and may be very painful. It is performed by, inserting a needle through the vagina and then into the uterus. Though now it is much widely done through the abdomen. Since this procedure actually takes samples from the placenta, it has been linked to deformities of the fetus, miscarriage and wrongful termination of the fetus through incorrect test results. Make sure you get a second opinion and perform amniocentesis before making any decisions on the condition of the embryo. It is usually performed between the 10th and 13th week of pregnancy. Make sure you have fully researched the doctor and facility performing this procedure.

CHAPTER FOUR

NO EXCUSES

When I found out I was pregnant, I immediately stopped drinking alcohol, and gave up my favorite source of fluids, Coca-Cola. Did I want to quit?? No, I did not and neither do you. But, I did and you will too. While you are the incubator to a pure, innocent baby, there will be many things you will not be able to do.
ABSOLUTELY NO EXCUSES!!!!

NO SMOKING- Smoking causes stunted fetal growth and development. Also, fetal distress, low birth weight, deformities, brain and spinal defects. Studies have shown carbon monoxide and nicotine in the umbilical cord, amniotic fluid, and your breast milk. You have a higher risk of having a premature or stillborn birth. You also increase your child's future to one of illness, learning disabilities, and the risk of SIDS during your baby's precious first months. Do I need to say more????

NO ALCOHOL- You may not have even one drink during your entire pregnancy; nor during the time you may breast-feed. Alcohol crosses into your child's bloodstream, and there is no amount safe enough to be absorbed by your developing baby. You increase your baby's risk of mental retardation, extreme facial and skeletal deformities, and death. Your child may also be born an "alcoholic", (fetal alcohol syndrome), and if lucky enough to have survived will go through symptoms of withdrawal. Your child will have learning deficiencies also to struggle with for life. Do not drink any alcohol when you are breast-feeding. I don't care what any expert tells you, in that it may be safe and may help to increase your milk supply. Do not believe this. The alcohol is absorbed into your breast-milk and therefore will be ingested by your growing baby. Can you possibly even think of having a drink now? If the answer is, "maybe", I will ask that you do not have a child right now and that you will not breast-feed either until you are ready to take full responsibility for every action you take that may harm your innocent baby.

NO ARTIFICIAL SWEETENERS: The chemicals in these sweeteners have been shown to cause cancer and fetal abnormalities. Though tests are still not 100% conclusive on the damage done to you and your unborn baby. I will strongly recommend that you do not consume anything that contains these sweeteners including:

Nutra Sweet
Aspartame, Acesulfame-K
Sweet 'n Low
Saccharin
Phenylalanine

NO CAFFEINE- Caffeine does cross the placenta and into your child's bloodstream. The problem with this is though it may not be harmful to you; your precious baby cannot filter the caffeine out of its

33

bloodstream. It therefore accumulates and this is where the damage may occur to your growing or breast-feeding infant. You also increase your risk of miscarriage and the chance of having a premature birth.

NO HERBAL TEAS CONTAINING- Black cohosh, blue cohosh, comfrey, dong quai, echinacea, ephedra, fenugreek, feverfew, garlic, ginger, pennyroyal, rosemary, safflower, saffron, sassafras, tansy, and willow bark. Some of these ingredients were used in previous centuries to promote a miscarriage in unwanted pregnancies. Two of these tansy and pennyroyal should be avoided at all costs. Do not take anything, in any form, containing any of these ingredients.

NO HAIR DYES (applied to scalp)- Because of numerous links of chemicals from hair dye being absorbed into your scalp and therefore found in your bloodstream, you are highly advised to forgo coloring. If you must color, talk to your colorist, who may be able to do highlights or foils to keep your hair color from fading. Just find any method that will not have color sitting right on your scalp.

NO NAIL POLSH- A recent study by the Environmental Working Group found that dibutyl phthalate or DBP; a chemical found in most nail polishes caused birth defects in lab animals. Do not take any chances. Get a white stick to make nails appear whiter and a buffer for shine. There are some nail polishes which do not contain this ingredient, so if you really need the polish check ingredient list carefully.

NO ALPHA-HYDROXY CREAMS- Any cream that is intended to penetrate your epidermis is not recommended by me during your pregnancy and if you are going to breast-feed. Why? This is just my extremism for caution due to the fact that these chemicals may pass into your bloodstream and therefore into your child's.

NO ASPIRIN OF ANY KIND (unless advised by your doctor)- Aspirin has been linked to extreme skeletal and facial abnormalities in laboratory mice. There has also been an increased risk of hemorrhaging to you and your baby, if you use aspirin during your last trimester. This hemorrhaging of your baby can lead to death. Do not take any aspirin if you have had a previous premature labor. The bleeding complications involved from aspirin consumption will not be a good factor in your baby's health due to a premature birth.

NO MEDICINE (unless advised by your doctor)- If you have to take any medicine make sure it is a life or death situation. Otherwise please refrain from taking ANY medicine at all. This includes over-the-counter medicines, any medicine you have currently been prescribed, and antibiotics. There has been one too many studies linking medication with fetal deformities. Do not take any chances, not even one pill, one time.

NO RETIN-A OR ANY OTHER TOPICAL MEDICATED CREAM (consult physician)- Any medicine that penetrates the epidermis and may enter your bloodstream is not advisable at this time. Do not use any acne or psoriasis creams or medications. There is a definitive link to birth defects.

NO ILLEGAL SUBSTANCES OR ANYTHING ELSE THAT YOU DO THAT MAY HARM YOUR UNBORN BABY- I do not think I even have to justify this with an explanation, but I will. Drugs cause birth defects, learning disabilities and DEATH. Your child will go through a severe withdrawal upon its premature birth. If it survives you will not only have the guilt to contend with but also a very sick, colicky, unresponsive, under-developed baby to care for every day of your already miserable life. Give your precious baby a chance; do not use drugs. Having a happy, healthy, and smiling baby in your arms will make such a world of difference in your life, you will be glad you gave up the drugs. You probably will never abuse your body again.

NO ANTACIDS-Studies are inconclusive. Do not use anything that is not 100% natural. You do not want any chemical in your system.

35

NO LAXATIVES-Though they have been shown to be safe. I myself will not use anything that enters my system and manipulates anything occurring naturally within my body. This has been shown to cross into your breast-milk and therefore into your child's. If you do not wish your child to have a laxative, do not consume one yourself. Remember what is in Mommy's system is in baby's system.

NO INSECT REPELLENTS (if you must use anything try Avon's Skin-So-Soft)- Insect repellents actually use insecticides to keep bugs at bay. These have been linked to cancer. I refuse to put insect repellent on myself or even my children to this day. Read the back of one of your insect repellents. Become aware.

You must also take a multi-vitamin and extra folic acid. I took a multi-vitamin made for women (GNC carries one, but you can also find excellent multi-vitamins for less at wholesale stores and other health stores), and an extra 800 mcg of folic acid daily.
I recommend taking your vitamins at night before you go to bed. They will be absorbed better since there are less frequent trips to the bathroom, also your body repairs itself at night and will use the vitamins more proficiently at this time. If you are experiencing nausea, it sometimes helps to take your vitamin at night. You may feel less sick at this time. Be sure to take your vitamins with either milk or orange juice. A thicker fluid helps the pills go down better and helps to eliminate the after taste some women find in their multi-vitamins.

Fact: Folic acid is imperative for the neural development of your unborn baby

I was given a prescription for prenatal vitamins, as do all pregnant women upon confirmation of their pregnancy. I never filled this prescription. I read all the ingredients listed on the insert and was surprised to find these prenatal vitamins contained a laxative. I believe in a complete pure system at this time and did not take them. Please read all ingredients on anything you are going to use at this time, prescribed or not. Question your doctor on everything and get his medical expertise on anything you will or won't be taking.

If you know you want to conceive, I urge you to begin taking care of yourself now. It is better for you and your child if you conceive while you are at your healthiest. Those first three months are vital for the development of your child. Most women don't find out they are pregnant well into their second month, and you do not want to have been abusing your body at this time. Trust me, you never want to look back and regret something you may or may not have done to help your unborn child.

Now, if you cannot do this for the few months it takes for your developing child to be born, you must seriously consider the fact that you are not ready for the enormous responsibility it takes to have a child. Remember no one is saying this is forever. As soon as your baby is born (and you are not breastfeeding) you can do whatever you want.

There are some other things that you may not be aware of that may put your developing baby at risk. I will list them:

LISTERIA- This bacteria lurks in foods like feta cheese and hot dogs (the water in the packaging is ideal for breeding). Though extremely rare this bacteria can cause your child to be born stillborn. I did not even touch a package of these for almost two years. Please consult your doctor and read as much as you can about Listeria. Be highly informed about everything concerning the health of your unborn child. You can read more on Listeria in The Pregnancy for Today's Woman, or the CDC.

X-RAYS- Avoid having any dental work or any kind of x-ray taken at this time, unless it is life and death. Low levels of radiation have been said to be safe, but tests still being done are inconclusive. Don't take any chances. I recommend not even standing by your microwave oven at this time. If possible don't use it at all, use the oven. You may think me extreme, but I took no chances with my developing precious baby. You may also want to avoid flying. There are higher levels of radiation as the plane gains altitude. You may insist if you must fly that you wish to be screened by a woman, so that you may avoid walking through the metal detector. This also goes for jails, courts, and some other state or security institutions.

SWIMMING- This is just totally my own extremism on safety. I never swam in a pool. I know that they recommend swimming as exercise, but the thought of inhaling the vapors of chlorine (which is a toxic chemical) and having chlorine saturated into my skin was something I could not do. My body incubates my innocent child and I would not ingest, breathe or have anything topical on my skin that I felt might be harmful to my child. I leave this one totally to your discretion. DO NOT DIVE OR SCUBA DIVE WHILE YOUR PREGNANT. DO NOT JUMP INTO POOL, IF YOU DO GO IN ONE.

CATS- If you have a cat, please arrange to have someone else clean up after your cat, especially its litter box. Cats fecal-matter contain a bacteria called Toxoplasma gondii, this may result in the pregnant woman contracting toxoplasmosis. This disease damages or kills the fetus in half of all occurrences. It is transmitted by moving the feces, and then by letting it become airborne, where it can be inhaled. When the cat litter is being disposed of, leave the room. If though, you have had this disease already, you are now immune and so will your fetus. You can have a blood test taken before you have even conceived to see if you have antibodies against this disease and are therefore immune. Testing done during pregnancy will detect the presence of antibodies, but not if they are old or new.
Please consult your doctor on this disease and get his advice about

testing yourself before you have even conceived if you do own a cat.

Other pets may be potentially harmful, by making you ill, though their effect will not harm your unborn child. Still be vigilant because any illness at this time may require antibiotics and not all can be used through your pregnancy, to cure you. You may want to wear gloves when handling any pet's feces. Also, you may want to take your pet to the veterinarian to ensure their health and yours.

Keep yourself healthy at this time, and ask for help with the care of animals at this time. It is only for a few months and it will be the difference for a lifetime of healthy children for you.

Please NO promiscuity. Life as we know it has changed no longer are carefree days and casual sex. Now comes STD's with no cure and AIDS which you can pass to your child and is a death sentence. Always be safe; know and trust your partner. As Grandma would say keep your shoulders back, head held high, and legs crossed truly makes a lady.....

The healthier you are, the healthier and stronger your child will be. I have only listed a few things for you to be cautious about. Please read other maternity books for more detailed information. I stress to you to think, and use common sense and logic for these nine months. If your gut reaction is that you feel it may not be in the best interest for your growing child, don't do it.

CHAPTER FIVE

LESS IS MORE

With pregnancy, comes some hard facts. You are going to gain weight, and your body will never be the same again. I am not saying that you won't still look just as good as you do now, but you will never have the same body, it may even be better, but not what it looks like today. Take lots of pictures to reminisce the glory of your pre-pregnant body.

Weight gain is vital for the health of your baby; do not diet EVER during these nine months. If you are going to consciously make an effort not to eat, so you do not put on weight, you are not ready to have a child. The first thing you must do as a mother is lose all selfishness in you. This means that you are going to put your child FIRST and if your body suffers a little extra wear and tear during these nine months, it was the first gift you gave your child. The gift at a chance for a very healthy future.

You must eat a balanced healthy blend of foods. Lots of milk and at least one glass of orange juice a day. Eat plenty of vegetables, fresh meats, fresh seafood, and give up fast foods at this time. Eat whatever you are craving, your body knows best what it needs right now. Try not to eat an entire gallon of ice cream a night if this is what you crave, and this goes for other foods. You are not dieting but we are not gorging ourselves with food at this time either. Eat until your satisfied, no more.

Make sure all your food is well cooked and fresh. If you are a vegetarian make sure your doctor knows. You may have to take extra supplements to ensure your child gets all of its nutrients. You will have to eat extra protein to make up for the lack of meat in your diet. Please read "What to Eat While Your Expecting" to help. I recommend everyone to read this book too.

I gained 40 – 50 pounds during each pregnancy. When the scale started reaching toward 180 by the last weeks of my pregnancy, I did not want to look at the scale any more. I ate very well during my nine months. I did most of my own cooking and very rarely ate out. I wanted to make sure that what I was eating was healthy and that all my food was well cooked. I could only know for sure, if I cooked it myself.

Most of the weight you put on will be from the baby, the rest from fluid retention, stored fat, and for most women and their partners, glorious huge breasts.

Most doctors recommend putting on 25 – 40 pounds as a standard weight gain for your pregnancy. Too little and too much is not good. Though, I met a blood technician who told me she put on 75 pounds during her pregnancy. One year later, she looked great and was back to pre-pregnancy weight, with a very healthy child. So, sometimes you can't always fit into a standard mold, your body and doctor will know what's best for you and your developing baby.

STANDARD WEIGHT GAIN:

41

Blood Volume- 4 lbs.

Breast T issue- 1-2 lbs.

Stored Fat- 4-? Lbs.

Fluid Retention- 4 lbs.

Baby- 6 – 9 lbs.

Uterus- 2 lbs.

Placenta- 1.5 lbs

Amniotic Fluid- 2 lbs.

During your pregnancy you will also not do any extreme exercise, or if possible none. That is right, no exercising, nothing, and none at all. I repeat, while you are pregnant maybe light meditative yoga geared for expectant moms or light weights for arms. During this time your body is constantly changing. You are going to get bigger – you do not want tight toned muscles at this time. You want a little relaxation of muscle and skin tone. I did not do any form of exercise while I was pregnant. Also, you never want to do anything that may harm your unborn child. Jiggling, exertion, and sweat are not worth in hindsight the little bit of muscle tone you are trying in vain to keep.

Spend this time relaxing and getting much needed sleep. If you wish to do some sort of exercise, you may walk. Walk at a normal pace. Stop and rest whenever you feel the least bit exhausted. You may walk, provided that you are with someone. If you are with your partner, let him hold your hand. If you are with a friend, keep them close to you. Do not walk at night, only during daylight. I insist on all these precautions in the event you fall, someone will be with you or hopefully prevent a fall from happening.

If you suffer from water- retention, as most pregnant women will, you will not even want to walk. You should rest as much as possible and drink plenty of fluids. Keep your feet elevated and lie down as much as possible. If you are pregnant during your last trimester and it is summer, stay in air- conditioned rooms as much as possible. Rest, rest, rest. This may be the last chance to sleep and lie down whenever you wish.

Another area of The Pod Method is to have no stress on your body at this time. I truly believe looser is better. It is easier for your child to come out if there is no resistance.

I gained a lot of weight during my pregnancy and did not exercise until I had completely stopped bleeding, which was about eight weeks. I will go into detail on this in a later chapter. I lost about 20 pounds in the first week after my child was born without even trying. I continued to lose weight as the weeks went by, but did not do any form of dieting until after I finished breastfeeding. I then went on a diet and took off the rest of the weight within three months. It takes about a year to get back to complete physical shape of your pre-pregnancy body.

Believe you will lose all your pregnancy weight fast and without effort. Constantly command your inner self to know that the weight is for your baby, and only for its health. You will put on as much weight as you must to ensure your child's health. You will know that this weight is for your child and will leave with the birth of your child. Every pound you gain during your pregnancy is for your child. It is not weight for you. It will go with the process of labor. Labor will trigger your body to begin losing all of your weight. Command your body that labor will be the trigger to start losing its weight. You must believe this and it will be so.

I lost almost 25 pounds within 3 days of giving birth. The rest of the weight continued to come off within months of the birth of my child. Since I breastfed my child I did not diet. This was to sustain the vitality and health of my milk. After I finished breastfeeding, I went on a diet and lost the last ten pounds that had not left due to the extra stores of fat your body retains on a breastfeeding mother.

I believed in letting my skin and body become looser so that tight toned muscles would not hinder the emergence of my baby during childbirth. I also believed that if my skin were looser it would be less prone to stretch marks. I never got any stretch marks during my two pregnancies. If your mother had stretch marks, it is usually believed that you will too. This is not true. My mother got a few stretch marks from her pregnancies and I never got any. I mixed together in my hands and slathered Nivea Lotion and St. Ives Collagen and Elastin all over my body after every shower. These creams helped keep my skin moisturized and supple. Though both of these creams, do not say they will prevent stretch marks, I did not get even one. Who knows?

I also did not get any varicose veins during my two pregnancies, and this is said to be hereditary related, too.

I believed I would not get them, and took care to make sure I would not. I shaved my legs and belly every day to naturally exfoliate (plus I hate the way hair looks on a pregnant woman's belly). If you are going to shave your belly, be extremely careful of your belly button.

I never wore panty hose, tight fitting shoes or clothes, which I believe is not good for your circulation. You do not want to wear anything constricting at this time on your body. I basically wore stretch pants and loose fitting tops my entire pregnancy. In the summer I wore loose cotton dresses. I wore NAOT sandals and shoes, which I believe

44

helped my entire body endure less stress. They are extremely comfortable and are made to fit the shape of your foot. I feel this helped my back, my legs and the non- occurrence of any varicose veins. Also, since my feet were so comfortable, it helped enormously with all this extra weight I had put on during my pregnancy.

SCIATICA- This lower back and leg pain may be one of the worse side effects from pregnancy. The best thing you can do is rest when this occurs. Sometimes it is just an odd position your child is in. Talk to your child and ask them to move their little body to a different position. Sometimes lying down on the opposite side may help the baby to shift its position. I only experienced this a few times. I asked my child to move and I rested. It usually went away in a matter of minutes. Do not bend or pick up heavy objects, this may aggravate it. Walking slowly may also help to ease the pain. Comfortable shoes are a must. Consult your doctor if this occurs a lot or is hindering your day- to- day lifestyle.

LEG CRAMPS- These painful spasms happen mostly at night. Straighten your legs and flex your ankles and toes, slowly toward your face. This should help. Some women have stated that standing on a cold surface helped to relieve their leg cramps. If this continues to occur, consult your doctor for the rare possibility that a blood clot may have formed in your vein.

BACKACHES- Back pain is probably going to occur, with all this extra weight on your belly. Try to stand straight. It may be hard towards the end, when you will be at your highest weight, and with a belly pulling you forward. Rest as much as possible. Do not stand or sit for long periods of time. Wear comfortable shoes and clothes.

STRETCH MARKS- These pink streaks on your body occur when the skin has stretched from the weight gain put on during your pregnancy. Do know that there are ways to minimize, but total prevention does not exist. If you do get stretch marks, they will fade as time goes by. If you are still unhappy consult a dermatologist. There have been excellent results with the removal of stretch marks with laser surgery.

VARICOSE VEINS- These broken blood vessels occur when excess weight and blood volume is intensified within your veins. These protruding veins or spider veins are unsightly and not something we would like to keep. They will subside after the birth of your child. If any have lingered and you are unhappy with them, consult your doctor. Varicose veins can be completely and safely removed now.

EDEMA- Water retention is probably the most hindering of side effects of pregnancy you can get. You have dealt with all the extra weight and to top it off, now you have bloated up so much you don't even recognize yourself. This happened to me during the hottest, humid summer I can remember with my first child. I recommend plenty of fluids and lots of rest. Air conditioning is a must. Try to get through this without medication. Consult your doctor on any swelling, as this symptom may be the underlying cause of preeclampsia (a form of high blood pressure). Do not stand for long periods. Do not wear any constricting clothes or shoes. Drink plenty of fluids.

You may also want to remove any rings or tight jewelry you wear by your third trimester. This is just a precaution in case you do experience swelling. You will not want your rings and especially your wedding band cut from your fingers because of the need to release pressure from the extreme swelling you may encounter.

CHAPTER SIX

TIGHTER THAN A DRUM

Recently, Kegel exercises have become very popular with pregnancy, and I will recommend that you do not do any during yours. Kegel's tone the vaginal and perineum muscles. I did not do even one Kegel during both my pregnancies.

I could not believe that anyone would want you to do Kegel exercises, especially at this time. Right now, you want as little resistance on your child's progress into this world. Tightening up the only way out is going to increase the time you spend in labor pushing. Also, the tighter you are the less the skin can stretch and the more stitches you will likely endure.

I completely believe this so much that I did not do any Kegel's after the birth of my first child because I knew I wanted another child and did not want to jeopardize the chances of my second child not making a speedy exit.

Now that I am finished with having any more children, I will do my pelvic toning Kegel's solely for my husband. Though he swears there is no difference in elasticity after our two children (smart man).

KEGEL-There are several different exercises that may be used to tighten the pelvic and perineum area. The easiest being to pretend you are stopping the flow of urination or preventing a bowel movement from occurring. Try it; you will feel the tightening of the muscles, there. Do this at least 100 times daily. Some women do this exercise while they are driving or talking on the phone.

Another Kegel exercise is a little more involved. It requires you to lie down on your back, head on a pillow. Bend your knees and place your feet about a foot apart. With arms resting at your sides, tighten up the muscles around your vagina and anus. Do about 25 repetitions four to five times.

Perform this exercise after you have finished having all the children you wish. This exercise will help to tighten and tone your vaginal area. Another benefit is that it helps strengthen the muscles surrounding a weak bladder.

CHAPTER SEVEN

AGAIN???????????????????????????????????????

In order to keep the vaginal muscles loose, supple, and stretched, you must have lots and lots of sex. I truly believe that this is the only way to keep yourself primed and ready for your child's exit.

Have you ever noticed that when you go without sex for a while, you tighten up and it takes a little work to loosen up the muscles of the vagina? Well, now is not the time you want to be tight. You will want your partner to keep you primed right up until your due date.

The more sex you have, the better. While having sex you can experiment by letting your partner find positions with you where he can have a 360-Degree thrust. This circular motion feels wonderful and will help to keep the opening stretched for your child to emerge through.

You will want your vagina as loose and supple as possible. I know that loose and supple is not how you want to think of your vagina, but you must. The vagina is the birth canal, the only way for your child to emerge naturally into this world. If you keep your vagina stretched during this time, your child will be able to emerge faster. When you are in the throes of labor, you will hope your vagina is loose enough to let your baby come right out, with no resistance.

When I was asked to push during labor, I was told I was doing it wrong. But, how could I know how to do it right? I never did this before. I was always told that when you are going to push, pretend you are going to the bathroom, having a bowel movement. You are then supposed to push down.

I believe most women have heard this too, and believe as I did to be true. When you push down pretending you are having a bowel movement, you are pushing with your sphincter muscle. This will not get your baby out.

No wonder so many women are scared to push, thinking if they do they are going to go the bathroom on their doctor! This alone can be why it takes so many women hours of pushing to get their child out. They are subconsciously fearful that if they do push, it will be the most embarrassing moment of their life. Also, they are probably pushing with the wrong muscle as I was.

As fast as my child emerged, less than ten minutes, I knew I could have helped to push him out even sooner. Since we have been pushing bowel movements out since we are born, it is no wonder that when someone says, "Push" we use our sphincter muscles, so that it will be second nature for you at the time of labor.

Recalling being told I was pushing wrong, I vowed I would not let this happen to me or to anyone else. If, I had known how to push before I went into labor, it would be one more childbirth empowerment tool I would have had.

I began to practice pushing and feeling where this muscle was while having sex. My husband never knew I was having more sex with him just so I could practice and stay primed for childbirth. My husband didn't mind having more sex and I don't think your partner will mind either.

Your partner will be of great assistance in helping you find the right muscles needed to push your child out during labor. While you are having sex, missionary style, you will practice.

While your partner has his penis inside of your vagina, you will be able to focus on the muscles of the birth canal. Now lift your legs up, knees bent, this will closely resemble the position you will be in while giving birth. With your partner's penis hard inside of your vagina, focus on the muscles surrounding his penis and push. Close your eyes and focus intently on your birth canal; now push down.

You will see that this is not the sphincter muscle. You can even practice pushing before you have even conceived. It is probably better to start practicing as soon as you know you want children. This is just in case your pregnancy is complicated and you are told from your doctor to refrain from having sex.

You will want to continue practicing as often as you can. Your goal is to be able to locate these muscles while not having sex. You want to be able to push forcefully when you are in labor. Knowing where the muscles are located to do this will help enormously when you are in labor.

Sexual relations may be terminated when:
1. You have experienced any unexplained bleeding
2. You have had, or are showing signs of miscarriage
3. If placenta previa exists (if your placenta has attached in the lower half of your uterus)
4. During your last trimester, if you have had or are experiencing signs of premature

51

labor.

5. Your water has broken (to ensure no foreign matter enters the amniotic sac, no sex!)

*Consult your doctor about this phase of The Pod Method. Make sure to get his or her authorization to proceed with this method. Let your doctor know immediately of anything you may feel worried or concerned about. If you experience pain or bleeding call your doctor immediately. Do NOT have sexual intercourse EVER!! if you are experiencing bleeding, pain, or cramps. Get your Doctors permission to continue having sexual intercourse. You may not be able to perform practicing this method for your entire pregnancy. PLEASE consult your physician on this chapter.

CHAPTER EIGHT

POWERFUL MIND   POWERFUL YOU

Ever since I was a child, I knew I wanted to have children. There was never a doubt in my mind that I would experience the joy of a baby and the pain of childbirth. It was during this time as a child, that I had heard the horror stories retold over and over again about 30 hour labors, hours of pushing and excruciating pain.

Since, I strongly knew I was going to have children, I vowed that would not be me. Yes, you say, you can vow all you want but there is absolutely nothing you can do. You see we have been told over and over again that there is nothing we can do, and that is where I truly believed "they" were wrong.

I was going to have a quick labor, yes I was, I truly believed. I know you are saying, "How? I cannot shorten my labor no matter what I do!" That is where you are very, very wrong. IT IS YOUR BODY, YOUR MIND.

You have an extremely powerful mind that controls all functions voluntary and involuntary. We have yet to tap into the full potential of the human mind. Yet, there are those who have had the courage to conquer what is known as impossible and triumph. There are masters of the mind who can slow their heartbeat until it stops. There are men and women who have healed themselves from terminal illnesses with the power of their minds.

The one thing that they all have in common is that they truly believed they could empower their being with complete control over their bodies. They truly believed in the power of the mind and with this power an awareness of themselves, and the power of control over their being. I will use the word believe often because you must, there can be no hesitation.

First you must believe you are strong, you are powerful. Repeat: I am strong; I am powerful. Repeat this constantly to yourself. You are not weak; you are not helpless. We were chosen to create life because we are strong and powerful. You will have to vanquish all thoughts that you have no control over your childbirth process.

Our bodies are designed to give life. Open your mind to believe your body will help you hasten the childbirth process.

You must be committed to a constant regiment of thought and actions from the time you find out you are expecting to your first thought of even wanting to conceive a child. If you know you are going to have children you can start preparing yourself mentally before you have even conceived.

As soon as you know you will want children you can start adapting to The Pod Method. I urge every woman to pass this book on to their daughters, so that they may have the knowledge to help them with the birth of your grandchild, one day. The sooner we as women can start empowering ourselves, the sooner we can take control of our lives. BELIEVE.

I will be giving you my most intimate of thoughts and actions. I will tell you everything I did during my pregnancy that led to a successful, rapid labor. Everything that I felt and believed were the reason I had a very easy labor, I have tried to relate to you as best I could. I hope to make you aware of why I did and may have thought a certain way so that you can understand and believe too without a shadow of doubt.

You must condition your mind to believe that you want a very quick labor. To begin this process you must first mentally visualize your due date. It is imperative that your due date is always in constant thought. This is the day when you will be looking forward to holding your baby in your arms. You will now always say to yourself, "I want my baby to be born right around this day." It is now your target date of empowerment. If you wish to think of a week before is fine, but do not ever think of a later date past your due date. I always told myself that I wanted my child to be born by this date; a week earlier would be fine, little one. I constantly talked to my child and let it know my wishes and to obey my inner commands.

Get a pregnancy calendar, fill it in starting from your due date and going backwards through the months till conception. Keep your doctor appointments, weight and any other statistics or information for you and your baby to cherish forever. Look at your calendar and due date often and repeat over and over to yourself that this is the day you want your child out – as quickly as possible.

Now, we all know that experts recommend talking to your unborn child. I believe this too. But, I believe in talking to your child and explaining what is occurring to him. Explain all the details of its conception and its impending birth. I knew my child would hear, learn, understand, and obey. I believed my talking to him would accomplish what I desired, a healthy, strong child, and a rapid labor.

I believed my child would hear my every word. I told my child that when it is time (your due date) you must help Mommy and get out fast, get out as fast as you can. Keep your head down, little one and get out as fast as you can. Repeat this to your child as many times daily as you can.

The object of this is to be in complete sync with your child and the task that lies ahead for both of you. Your due date will be a constant focus for you and your child. Your child will sense and know when this date nears, and will be ready to do as his Mommy asked.

Telling your child to keep his head down is very important. You want a natural delivery. If your child is in a breech position (which is legs first), most often than not you will end up with a C-section. Your doctor will try to turn your child, and sometimes the child will turn on its own. But why take any chances. Talk to your child and ask it to keep its head down. It will obey your commands. My children were both head down by my second trimester in my pregnancy. They were prepared very early to make their journey into my arms.

Another aspect of talking to your child is when you are alone. This is a most joyous time for you to completely enjoy your child and the special bond that only the two of you share.

When you are alone, lay down with your hands on your belly. Close your eyes and focus intently on your child floating peacefully within your womb. Go to your child and smile, your child will smile back. Embrace your child and tell it to grow strong and healthy. Tell your child that a very special day will be arriving (your due date) soon. Tell your baby, "Mommy will tell you when this day is near." " I need your help, little one, you will have to keep your head down and come out as fast as you can when this day arrives."

Now lock minds with yours and your baby. Show your baby the way out. Head down and through your cervix into the birth canal and out. Tell your baby not to be scared, "Mommy is always here."

In my opinion, your child will hear you and will help you when you are in labor. You must believe this. Your child can sense and feel all your thoughts and emotions, as it co-exists within you. If you believe

56

this and tell your child from the time it was conceived, it will hear you and do as Mommy wishes. Tell your child often to grow strong, healthy, and that you cannot wait to hold them in your arms. Believe your baby can hear and sense your wishes. BELIEVE.

You have talked to your child and there will be more that your child will learn from you with The Pod Method. But now you must take a deep look into yourself and know of some phrases or thoughts that may also hinder a rapid birth of your child.

I never said, "I love being pregnant!" I would hear expectant mothers say this and I would cringe. Who wants to gain weight? Not me! I never loved being pregnant. What I loved was the end result my pregnancy was going to bring me. What I loved and the only thing I was going to love, was my child in my arms.

I truly believe that if you constantly say you love being pregnant your mind begins to believe this too. You have now conditioned your mind to believe that pregnant with the baby inside of you is what makes you most happy. So, after months of being so happy pregnant, your mind and body are not going to want to let your baby go. You have just spent nine months saying, "This is what I love and want, being pregnant."

Is it any wonder that after this kind of self- brainwashing, your body now believes what it has been told. On a subconscious level your body truly believes, that you want to stay pregnant. You control your mind and body for good or worse. It can be for positive or negative. To hinder or help you at a time of great need. This is not a time you want any thought conscious or not to betray you by delaying your labor.

Most women can halt their labors from sheer will and fear. That is how powerful the mind is. Their bodies will fight this childbirth from happening, because then technically they will then not be pregnant anymore. If you train your mind and body to believe pregnant is what you most desire, you will be making a very big error, in judgment. Your labor will be long and painful due to the fact that you conditioned your mind to believe it is the baby IN you that makes you happy. This is a major mistake.

You are not in love with being pregnant. You are in love with the baby you are going to have. Never say, "I love being pregnant." Say, "I can't wait until my child is in my arms."

This subconscious thought of always being pregnant. Stems from a male dominated world that loves their women barefoot, pregnant, and in the kitchen. We have all heard this saying, and in an indirect way we too, think we want to always be pregnant, for then we are more loved in this condition.

Do you feel that people are nicer to you, especially your partner? It is common for most women to start associating a change in attitudes attributed to being a pregnant woman. Do not let yourself start believing that this condition is going to change your life. Being pregnant does not change your life, your baby in your arms does. You must keep a constant focus on your child. You must keep a constant focus on your child. Your baby in your arms is going to give you the most joy. Nothing else comes close to this. People are nice to you because of your beautiful smile. Your partner is nice to you because he loves you.

We are pregnant for one reason only, to create life, and to smile down upon our beautiful baby. We will endure the process of pregnancy to achieve this goal.

Now that you have begun the process of mentally controlling the process of childbirth, you will now visually control the process. Using visual stimuli will help you to see your goal. It will help in your quest to achieve your goal of a rapid labor.

When you reached the onset of labor you will be hoping for your cervix to dilate from one to ten centimeters. You will learn from your readings that your baby will not come out until you are fully dilated. This is your ultimate goal and what you must truly believe will happen quickly. This is your most important step, dilating your cervix. I will tell you how I discovered The Pod Method Visual Tool, and how you will use it for your own pregnancy.

At the time of my first child, I was living in a basement apartment, which my husband had built. He will never know how much he helped visually condition my mind to believe.

I knew in order to have a rapid labor I must dilate my cervix as fast as I could. How to do this was my dilemma. I mentally started the process of commanding my body to obey. When one day I looked up. This changed the course of my making a rapid labor attainable. I now knew without a shadow of a doubt what I saw would also help visually command my mind and body to obey. I believed and knew a rapid labor was going to happen.

My husband had installed recessed lighting in the ceiling. It amazed me how much it looked like the head of my baby coming out of my cervix.

I began staring at the recessed lighting everyday (lights dimmed or off) and would believe this was my cervix and my child. The recessed lights were round and approximately ten centimeters in diameter; this was my cervix. The halogen light bulb in my mind was the head emerging from my cervix and vagina. I concentrated on this image every day.

My desire was to mentally command my cervix to dilate rapidly. To do this, I knew I had to go from one to ten centimeters dilation. Visually focusing and mentally commanding within, I said, "One, Two, Three, Four, Five, Six, Seven, Eight, Nine, Ten, One to Ten, cervix open as fast as you can, one to ten as fast as you can, OPEN, OPEN, cervix as fast as you can", willing my cervix to dilate quickly.

The light you remember; was the baby's head. I would imagine it was my baby emerging from my cervix. I would then close my eyes and talk to my child. I would concentrate on my child and tell it to help me. I would tell my child, "Get out as fast as you can, help Mommy, help Mommy little one and get out, so Mommy can hold you in her arms." I repeated this constantly myself, several times a day. Visually and mentally I believed.

If your cervix does not dilate fully you will not be able to have a vaginal delivery. If your cervix is taking too long to open, your doctor may not let you have a vaginal delivery (due to the fact of extra stress put on your baby in excessively long labors).

You want your cervix to dilate rapidly. This is the most important strength of will you must command your body to do. You will spend as much time as you can focusing on The Pod Method Visualization Tool.

I designed The PMVT to resemble the recessed lighting in my own home. You will envision that the outer black circle is your cervix; the yellow circle is the head of your baby. The outer ring of the black circle is ten centimeters. The blackness surrounding the head of your baby is the birth canal, from which your baby will emerge.

You will think words like roomy and cavernous, whenever you think of your child emerging from your birth canal.

The birth canal is from your cervix to your vagina. I always mentally and visually focused on the word cavernous. It meant huge, open space, and endless depth. I knew in order for my child to emerge, he first had to squish through the birth canal. If I mentally and visually believed my birth canal was cavernous, then this meant my child had plenty of room from which to emerge. He would literally come right out as soon as my cervix was fully dilated and I gave one push.

Always use the image of cavernous when you think of your birth canal.

Now mentally focus on The PMVT, look deep within it and in yourself. Think of your due date, this is when you will go into labor. This is when you want your body to obey your command to open your cervix rapidly. You will now prepare your mind and body for this to occur as you wish.

Repeat over and over to yourself daily the following as you look at The PMVT:

One, Two, Three, Four, Five, Six, Seven, Eight, Nine, Ten, OPEN, OPEN, cervix as fast as you can, OPEN as fast as you can, Open as fast as you can, OPEN.

Mentally visualize your cervix opening and the head of your baby emerging. Tell your child to help you. Close your eyes and focus on your child.

Say, "Help me, little one, help Mommy and get out, Mommy wants to hold you, keep your head down and when Mommy tells you to come out (your due date) help me."

I truly believed I could will my body with the power of my mind to accelerate my cervix dilating. I knew if I could do this, I would have a rapid labor and endure less pain. The shorter the labor the less pain you will have to endure.

By mentally preparing my cervix to open rapidly, I knew it would take hours off of my labor. If you focus and command your body to do as you wish, you will also be able to take hours off of your labor.

61

Remember, each delivery will be unique. But even one hour or one minute less is a blessing when you are in labor.

This is one of the most important steps of The Pod Method. I believe this was the main reason my labor was a rapid success. This form of auto-suggestion of the mind, has been used for years to help people attain desired results they felt they would not attain otherwise. By constantly repeating a phrase over and over again you are transforming your complete thought process to believe that this is truth.

If you believe everything you say and do as truth your mind and body will too. You are the commander of your body. You can lead your mind and body down a path of complete awareness and it will then do as you wish. This is a very important realization that you really do have the power to alter and make things happen within your body. The human body is an amazing creation and capable of performing many wonderful feats.

Your pregnancy is one of these miracles and your body is capable of listening to your wants and needs and performing them at your will. The Pod Method steps may seem outrageous to some. But these steps have been designed with one mission in mind: To help you have a very easy labor. You must have your mind completely aware of the process it will be going through and so should you, if you wish to be in complete control.

By looking at The PMVT you are actually seeing for yourself and so is your mind what your cervix must do. You must believe this is your cervix and connect your mind and body as one to believe you will dilate rapidly and your baby will emerge as quickly as possible.

This is why you must keep The PMVT in visual sight as much as possible. You want to constantly be aware of your cervix and what it must do. When you go into labor your mind, body, and cervix will only know that it is to do as you have taught it. Your mind and body will enforce this Pod Method education you have given it and help your cervix to dilate rapidly.

After nine months of you concentrating on The PMVT as your cervix, your body will not even have any notion that it is not supposed to take days and excessive hours to dilate.   Your cervix will now after nine months only know and believe one thing as you go into labor; it must dilate rapidly.

I urge you to do this exercise every day, from the onset of knowing you are pregnant. Keep The PMVT in a place where you spend most of your time. Make sure to keep constant focus on your cervix. It will open rapidly. Keep constant focus on your child. Your child will help you and emerge swiftly, safely, and healthy.
BELIEVE.

CHAPTER NINE

GO AWAY

Now that you have mastered most of The Pod Method steps to having a quick labor, you will learn one of the most vital steps you need most. Pain control is probably the one method you will use and hope works the best. If you can master your pain, you will have one more empowerment tool to help you in your quest for achieving a natural labor.

There are many different childbirth methods that you will learn about and want to use for your labor. Most of these methods will help immensely. The difference between The Pod Method and other methods is that you have to be consciously aware of your actions, whereas with The Pod Method your entire being has been conditioned to automatically subconsciously take over for you and allow your body to have an easier labor.

When you are in labor you will endure a pain so great that no matter what childbirth methods you have learned they may not be able to help you during your time of greatest need. When you begin to experience pain during your contractions you may not be able to do anything but focus on the pain. Depending on your tolerance for pain is a major factor in the delivery of your child.

If this is your first child, nothing and no one can help you relate to the pain you will experience during labor. Each person's threshold for pain is different. Some may be able to tolerate pain better than other's. I will tell you that the pain was greater than anything I could have imagined. But, the main thing was that it was happening to ME. I had to do what I felt would help me tolerate and continue a natural childbirth with the least pain.

When you begin to have contractions they will become stronger and more painful with each progressive one. You may be in a complete shock when this occurs. No matter what you have done to educate yourself it may not prepare you for the pain you will experience during your contractions.

It is such an intense pain that I personally was not able to use one of the most highly regarded methods, Lamaze. I did not do my breathing exercises as I was taught.

During my labor, I must have stopped focusing on just breathing. I was so intent upon willing the pain away, that a nurse told me to breath. My husband held my hand and counted as we had been taught in our Lamaze classes together. Though I just breathed normally, not the way I had been taught from Lamaze. I do feel my husband helped me by keeping me focused on just the act of breathing. You may hold your breath as I had begun to do. He did in fact help me to breathe easier, by his counting; I was now aware of the fact that I must breathe even if it was not exactly as I had been taught from Lamaze. Lamaze will also be invaluable to you too. I did not use the Lamaze breathing method, because all I could do was focus on willing the pain away, I was unable to focus directly on my breathing methods or to count how many breaths I was taking during my contractions.

65

I do so stress that you learn every childbirth method you can. Each pregnancy and woman is unique. You may find that the Lamaze or another method will be of great help during the birth of your child.

Every woman's body is designed differently. Some woman may be looser or tighter, wider or narrower. This unique design of each woman should not hinder your labor. The female body is still genetically designed to give birth and will allow the process to happen swiftly.

The weight of your child should also not hinder its labor. Though a six- pound baby may seem that it should come out easier, this is no guarantee. Your internal organs were designed to stretch enough to allow room for your child to emerge swiftly. A pound or two will not make a whole lot of difference when you are in labor. Please do not stop eating or ask to be induced early so that you might have an easier labor by delivering a baby who may weigh less. This is a ridiculous myth and dangerous to the health of your child.

What The Pod Method of pain control will do is help your mind and body obey command words that will trigger de-sensitivity to the pain you will endure. You will still be experiencing the pain, but you will seem as if your body is feeling this pain on a different dimension. I know this sounds completely strange. But, any person who has endured a terrible pain put upon their bodies for a long or short period of time will tell you that they finally "detached" from the pain and was able to endure it to the point where it was gone.

This detachment to pain is a way of your mind and body protecting itself. You have probably experienced this effect at least once in your life. It occurs when you let yourself be "absorbed" into the pain. You will reach a level of calmness to focus on your pain and allow your-self to be soothed and protected by this trigger mechanism.

When I was in labor and the intensity of contractions started to occur and with it bringing on intense pain, I could only focus on bringing this mechanism in to play to protect me. I knew I had to endure the pain if I wanted a natural labor. I wanted no drugs of any kind in my system and to do this I had to be able to tolerate the pain.

This trigger mechanism protected me and I was able to have a natural delivery without any drugs. Also, the use of all the other steps from The Pod Method combined enabled an overall complete process of a rapid labor. This Pod Method step will be a determining factor in the success of having a natural labor with no drugs. If you are as determined as I was, and other woman to forgo drugs you will find this step of great reassurance because it does work.

I will now tell you in a little greater detail how my labor's progressed and what this trigger mechanism is.

As you know, I was petrified of having a long and painful labor that I began the process of controlling and preparing my body for the momentous task of a quick delivery. I mentally and visually commanded my body to obey my wishes and there was not one shred of doubt once I began.

If I did not completely believe I could shorten the childbirth process there was the chance that subconsciously I could prolong it. I had total faith in my body and that of my unborn child, in that he would help me and emerge quickly. I completely believed and you must too.

I am 5'7, I weigh about 130 pounds and have no medical history that could have hindered my use of The Pod Method. Mine was a very uncomplicated normal pregnancy.

I spent months visually and mentally preparing myself for this day, and it arrived with a splash. My water broke around 5:30pm on July 21st, one week before my due date (call your doctor immediately when your water has broken). I got to the hospital around 6pm.

Dr. Wider checked me and said that my cervix wasn't even two centimeters dilated. Dr. Wider then told me, because my water had broken, they would most likely induce me in the morning, and I would deliver then.

It is extremely rare for any woman whose water has broken and not even two centimeters to dilate to 10 centimeters in less than three hours. Statistically this just does not happen.

Once your water breaks, your OBGYN will want your child out as quickly as possible, usually within 48 hours at maximum. This is due to the fact of your baby losing amniotic fluid to protect it and the greater chance of infection due to the fact air and foreign bodies can now enter your uterus.

I completely do not believe in being induced. I know so many woman who have had this done to them, and did not have a successful natural labor. First off, when you are induced it is no guarantee your cervix will dilate. Secondly, your contractions are so intense and powerful due to the drug, Oxytocin that you will most likely request an epidural to get you through this.

I know so many women who were induced, then left for almost 20 hours to suffer with excruciating contractions. They not only had to use drugs in which they were so against in the birth of their child, they were then told they could not even have a natural labor due to the fact their cervix still hadn't dilated enough. These poor women were given C-sections. I think this is atrocious. Not only, did they have to suffer intense contractions, and have an epidural just to be able to relax and get some much- needed sleep, they ended up with C-sections.

If at all possible, discuss with your physician if he will work with you in delaying any form of drugs to induce you. Just because you are induced does not guarantee your cervix will dilate sufficiently. Do though heed any advice from your doctor especially if it is for the health and wellbeing of your child. If this is your only option, you must comply with your doctor. The end result of a healthy, beautiful baby in your arms is your only goal. How you have to achieve this goal does not matter in the least.

Well, back to my story. Dr. Wider left believing I would not deliver that night. I knew differently. I had been preparing myself for this moment and now my body was shifting into gear and beginning to obey all my commands I had communed within myself these past nine months.

I told the nurse that my contractions were extremely powerful, and that I had to be having the baby now. She told me to relax, that I would probably have a long night and to try and rest. I begged the nurse to check me again because my contractions were so intense. She must have heard in my voice, a certain octave that comes with a woman in the late stages of your labor.

I will be honest in that this was the only time I felt a slight tinge of fear. This was my first child. I knew I was experiencing intense contractions. If my contractions were this painful and powerful at two centimeters, how could I endure the contractions at five or six centimeters? I asked the nurse to please check me again.

The nurse checked my cervix. She told me I was about five or six centimeters. I was relieved and now totally sure that my labor was progressing rapidly. I knew I could endure the pain; I was halfway there, in such a short time.

She then asked me if I wanted Demoral, or an epidural, to which I refused both pain medications. She asked me two times if I was sure I did not want any drugs. She said I should take the Demoral, it would take the edge off. I asked her if it would take the pain away. She said,

"No, it will only take the edge off."

I told her all I wanted was for the pain to "go away". I thought to myself what exactly does taking the edge off. It would probably make me feel lightheaded and distract me and my mind and body from the process of helping me have a rapid delivery. Also, how long would it last? Definitely not long enough, and now I had destroyed nine months of a total pure system for my child.

I refused to put drugs into my system and into my child's. I don't care what they tell you, that it will not reach your child's system. How can this be 100% true? Something has to reach my child. After all, I am its life. What is in my body will eventually pass into my child's. I completely believe this true.

I did not come all these months making sure my child's system was pure to now drug him up moments before his entry into this world. My innocent child whom I had ensured every day of his life with total health and love was going to stay without any foreign chemicals in his system. I was determined and prepared.

I will say that the pain is so intense and powerful, that if your labor is not progressing rapidly and you need the drugs to sustain you during your labor, I would not blame you at all. Do not feel guilty or feel like you failed your child if you do ask for pain medication during the birth of your child.

As I have said, "Every woman's threshold for pain is different." No one is feeling your pain, but YOU. If it is more than you can bear, take the drugs. They are available and will help you. I do hope that if you mastered all the steps of The Pod Method, you will never have to make this difficult choice, especially if you and your partner were set on having a complete natural delivery, without drugs. If you have conditioned your mind and body, your labor will progress swiftly enough that your body can and will endure the pain of childbirth,

70

without the need for pain medication

My cervix went from one to ten centimeters dilation in less than three hours. I recall Dr. Wider in total amazement at the door, pulling his surgical gloves on as quickly as he could. The nurses were yelling at me not to push, that I had to wait for the doctor. Let me tell you, there is no waiting for anyone. If anyone ever tells you not to push and you can stop pushing, I would love to know how you did this. You must have an amazing willpower to stop pushing when your child is coming down the birth canal. I kept pushing. Stopping the process went against everything I had trained my body to obey.

I pushed less than ten minutes and my child emerged into the world at 9:01 pm. He was 8lbs. 4oz. and 20 inches long. My beautiful angel was here. Healthy, alert, and pink skin tone. He was perfect, and already trying to lift his head to see his Mama and Dada and opening his eyes and hands. Amazing.

I did not have an episiotomy. I did not want one, and was so relieved that I had a great doctor who cared about my wishes. Also, I think the fact that my pregnancy was progressing so swiftly; there really wasn't any time or reason to perform this procedure.

I needed about three stitches, which were never of any consequence. The cuts were so tiny that the three stitches were mostly a precaution to ensure that my bleeding was completely stopped. Even the tiniest cut will most probably be stitched at this time to ensure you are not experiencing any complications. They will clean you up and make sure that the bleeding has stopped and is just the normal afterbirth bleeding that you will now have for about two months.

The stitches were never any bother. I experienced absolutely no pain from them or burning when I went to the bathroom. I was mildly sore, down there, but never took any pain medication, not even aspirin. I refused the ice pack most women hold between their legs after giving birth due to hours of intense pushing. I totally did not need it and just found it cold and annoying. I thanked the nurse and told her I really did not need the ice pack anyway.

I never even used the topical medicated pain cream that hospitals provide you, for I knew I wanted to breast feed and still wanted a pure system.

During my labor the pain was worse than anything I had ever experienced. I was shocked at how intense and deep within my being the pain delved into. It is such an intense pain, that I was grateful my labor progressed so fast. I went without pain medication. But, if I would have had to endure this pain for twenty or more hours, I don't know if I could have done without.

I commend and salute all those mothers who did endure and forgo drugs during excessively long labors. Though I had so completely prepared myself for this moment, it is still a shock to your system once the intensity of your contractions start. I am so grateful that The Pod Method worked to such a success, that I was able to allow my body to take over and help me. That is why The Pod Method is so vital to know. You have commanded and trained your body to such an extent that even if you go into a "shock" from the pain, your body will trigger all of its defenses you have taught it and continue to help you have a rapid, easy labor with minimal pain.

I had gone to Lamaze classes to learn their breathing techniques to use while I was in labor. I never used them. It took all my power to concentrate on willing the pain away. I could do nothing else.

My labor had progressed so rapidly that I could not use the Lamaze method. The Lamaze method is instrumental in helping labors that are not progressing quickly. It will help you keep focused on what you are doing and help to keep you from hyperventilating during the long duration between your childbirth stages. Though the Lamaze method may help you even with a very rapid labor also. We are all individuals. Though I did not use this breathing method, you may. You will be thankful to know the Lamaze method if you come to a point during your labor where it will help you immensely.

With use of The Pod Method, your labor will go from one stage to the next so rapidly, that you may not have the chance to worry about your breathing technique. I still believe it is vital for you to learn the Lamaze breathing method. You may or may not need it, but it doesn't hurt to be fully educated on different childbirth methods.

During my pregnancy, I knew that there was going to be pain involved during my labor. This is another reason why I developed The Pod Method.

The faster my labor progressed the faster the pain would go away. But, even with a very fast labor there would still be enormous pain involved. I knew to get through this without any pain medication I had to prepare myself, and you must too.

First, remove all fear that you may have about the pain you feel you may experience. Fear is your enemy.

Close your eyes and reach deep within yourself. Go to a place deep within your mind, a place where all is calm. Now imagine you are in labor and the pain is starting to intensify. Tell your mind to make the pain go away. Visualize yourself in labor and the pain ebbing away. Like a beautiful clear blue stream flowing away. As the water gently flows away, so does your pain.

Command your body to make the pain "Go Away". You want your entire being to know that when you begin to experience labor, certain things will occur to your body. You want your mind and body so well trained and prepared, that you do not have to make a conscious effort for your body to obey your commands. It is imperative to the success of a rapid, less painful labor that you believe and have mastered all of The Pod Method steps.

Command your body to make the pain "Go Away". You can practice this technique as often as you can. What you will want to happen while you are in labor is for the words, "Go Away" to trigger this calming effect.

When you are in labor you will only experience pain during your contractions. As soon as the contraction is gone, so is the pain. You will know your cervix is dilating by the intensity of your contractions. Your contractions will become stronger and stronger as your cervix dilates.

When you feel the contraction coming, hold onto your partner. Move into any position you feel more comfortable in. I will tell you that when you are at the very end of your labor you will be limited to your movements by the nurses or doctor. This is because they will want you in a "safe" position for the arrival of your child.

Focus on the pain and say, "GO AWAY". Repeat this over and over again to yourself. You do not have to even speak it aloud, though I did once and had to apologize to my doctor by telling her that I did not want, " her to go away", just the pain. You can mentally command within your mind when you say, "Go Away".

You do not want the contractions to go away, just the pain. The contractions are going to bring your beautiful baby to you. Tell the pain to "GO AWAY". When your baby is in your arms, trust me there will be no more pain. It is all gone, completely, instantly gone. Believe you can make the pain go away. You can command your body to obey your wishes.
BELIEVE.

Since, I knew I was going to have another child, I continued my use of

The Pod Method. I found out I was pregnant nine months later. I again was petrified of a long and painful labor. I knew statistically that your second labor is faster, but each pregnancy is unique. I put fear out of my mind and visually and mentally commanded my body to get this baby out even faster with no pain whatsoever. I truly believed my baby and I would accomplish this.

My second child was born nine days before my due date. She arrived January 9th at 6:34 AM. She was 8lbs. 7oz. and 21 inches long. My entire labor was one hour and thirty-four minutes.

My contractions started at around 5 AM, and were four minutes apart (call your doctor when your contractions are about five minutes apart). I got to the hospital at 6 AM. My husband was frantic as soon as I woke him up to tell him I was having contractions. He knew how fast my first labor was and that I had continued the use of The Pod Method. He had visions of pulling over and having to deliver our child in our car.

Dr. Marin was waiting for me and ushered me right in to the birthing room. She knew about my history with my first child's rapid birth. She then told the nurses I would labor quickly. She broke my water and told me I was progressing so rapidly that I was going to deliver in minutes.

I said, "Go Away" to the pain as soon as my contractions became more intense. I truly believe that two years of preparing my mind abolished all pain. I was incredulous that I was going to deliver my child any minute since I felt absolutely no pain. I honestly only had one contraction that was painful and even that one was nothing.

When Dr. Marin told me my baby's head was here, I gave one push and my perfect, beautiful princess; alert and healthy emerged. It was thirty- four minutes since I had gotten to the hospital. I again had not had an episiotomy. I was again given three stitches, which were never of any consequence. I was not sore at all and felt so great; I had to pinch myself that this just really happened so quickly.

Everyone tells me that I should have lots of children since I delivered so easily. It was my intense fear of going through a long and painful labor that I developed this method. I truly believed and I had a three and a half hour labor with minimal pain with my first child, and a one and a half hour labor with absolutely no pain for my second child after faithfully using The Pod Method now for two years.

Yes, I did have wonderful labors and no I do not want any more children. Just because my labors were easy does not mean I want a "Brady Bunch Family". This will soon be the norm for all women, fast, easy, and less painful labors. Whether you have one or ten. No woman will ever have to suffer the consequences of a long and painful childbirth. Childbirth will never again be associated with fear and pain, but only one of complete ease and joy.

I believed and you must too.
BELIEVE.

I will tell you of some different forms of pain medication used today in the process of delivering your child without pain. I highly urge you to consider the fact that whatever goes into your system will ultimately end up in your child's. I know childbirth is painful, but do you really want these drugs in your pure innocent child's? I ask you to really try to forgo any drugs during your labor. You can do it!

HYPNOSIS-This form of reducing pain during childbirth has become very popular in the past few years. You will go to a hypnotist for several sessions. You will then be given a tape to listen to while you are in labor. I know many women who said this helped them to alleviate the pain.

DEMORAL-This drug is one of the most popular to be given to the mother in pain. It diminishes the pain, though not completely. This drug is morphine, which is a narcotic. It has been linked to increased fetal heart distress. Traces of this drug and others like it have been found in the mother's breast milk after giving birth. If you plan on breast-feeding I highly encourage you not to use this or any other drug during the birth of your child. If you still feel you need some form of this type of pain reliever do not give your child your first or even second batch of breast milk. Pump and dispose of your breast milk. Though this is an extreme shame because your first milk you produce is colostrum, which is highly rich in proteins and antibodies and is vital for the health of your child. This is why I urge you not to use this or any other drug especially if you want to breast-feed.

There are a variety of drugs under many different names, which may be offered to you if request relief. I would be wary of the newer ones because tests are still ongoing and not conclusive. This meaning; these drugs potential harmful side effects have yet to be substantiated. I would not even want the drugs, which have been around for years. They have been seen to cause potential side effects to the mother (nausea) and to your child (fetal heart distress). Why take any chances.

EPIDURAL or SPINAL BLOCK- This form of drug relief is now the most common one used and asked for by laboring women. They both involve inserting a long needle into your spine. The spinal block actually passes into your spinal column, while the epidural only touches the surface. Both of these drugs give instantaneous relief.

This procedure numbs you from the waist down. You may not be able to bear down during the final stage of labor. This effect may prolong the birth of your child, since you may not be able to forcefully push when needed. Though it is stated that an epidural effects are less severe and you may be able to do some pushing.

If you have a spinal block you will have this procedure performed whenever you begin to feel the effects wearing off. This may be performed several times before you deliver your child.

If you have an epidural they will probably administer a catheter, which will continually administer the drug at intervals to keep you free from pain.

EPISIOTOMY-This procedure is becoming quickly a thing of the past. Doctors are finding that the drawbacks to this procedure are far more than once thought. Episiotomy is the cutting of your perineum area. This is the area from your vagina to your rectum. It is believed that by doing this procedure you will incur less tearing and your child will be able to come out faster.

This is totally false. There is no evidence that you will incur less tearing. You still may tear even with an episiotomy and it may be worse due to the severe cut your doctor has just given you.

Discuss the performance of an episiotomy before you are in labor with your doctor. Find out what they are most likely to do to you while you are in labor. If you do not wish this procedure done tell your doctor before you are in the birthing room. This way you can get all the facts from him or her. You can have all your questions answered and you can stress that you do not want an episiotomy.

When you are in labor tell your doctor again that you do not want an episiotomy. Tell your doctor that only if there is any risk to your child, will you have this procedure performed. Each labor is unique, and it may be necessary for your doctor to perform this procedure. Ninety percent of all pregnancies are normal and routine. If you fall into an uncomplicated labor percentage you can express fiercely that you do not want this procedure done. If for any reason your child's life and health may be at risk, then this procedure will be imminent and you will surely approve of having it done.

If you are going to have an episiotomy performed, this will be the only time I will urge you to get a local anesthetic. This procedure is extremely painful and you will need anesthetic for when the cut is performed and for when the stitches are put in after the birth of your child.

There are two different forms of local anesthetic used for this procedure, lidocaine and chloroprocaine. If at all possible ask for the latter, which may fall under the name of Nesacaine. This one has been shown to have the smallest, if any levels of this drug to enter into your child's bloodstream.

The stitches used during this procedure dissolve within a week. You will not have to worry about going back to your physician to have them removed.

OXYTOCIN- This drug usually dispensed as "Pitocin" is used to induce labor. This drug is the same as the oxytocin, which is released in a woman's system naturally during the onset of labor. This should never be performed just for the sake of getting your baby out because you or your doctor just can't wait for nature to take its course.

This drug produces very hard and prolonged contractions. It affects your baby to such extreme; that in 90% of induced labors you will be given a C-section because of your baby going into fetal distress.

Because your contractions are now drug induced and so powerful, oxygen levels are not adequately sustained within your blood. Thus, affecting your baby and putting it at risk.

You will, if given this drug have to have an epidural for pain relief. Your contractions brought on by this drug are so powerfully strong and intense that you will not be able to forgo drugs.

79

This inducing of labor is most often done if your water has broken and the onset of labor has not begun within twenty-four hours at the very most. If your water has broken, amniotic fluid has begun to diminish within the placenta. Also, the entering of foreign bodies into the uterus is very likely. To make sure there is no risk of infection to you or your baby, you will be induced.

If you have any medical conditions like hypertension, kidney disease or diabetes, your doctor may talk with you about the possibility of having to induce you. This is to keep you from an overdue baby and putting any more stress upon your body.

There are some risks associated with inducing labor. Please talk to your physician about every aspect of this procedure. Some risks are: ruptured uterus, fetal distress, injuries to your baby, and very rarely death of the baby. I do stress that it is EXTREMELY rare for any harm to come to your child with this procedure. But please be aware of all the risks.

If your doctor calls for an emergency C-section, which will be highly likely with this drug, do not hesitate in having the C-section done. Get your baby out and into your arms as quickly as you can.

If you have had a previous C-section, or have any contagious infectious disease of the genital area, do not have this procedure done. If you have multiple fetuses or placenta previa, again, do not have this procedure performed.

There are many circumstances, which may occur, leading up to the birth of your child. Your only mission is the arrival of your baby safely in your arms. Just please be informed about everything concerning you and your baby. Remember your doctor is the only one who knows what is best for you and your baby.

CHAPTER TEN

HAPPY HEALTHY YOU, HAPPY HEALTHY BABY

I'm sitting here typing, while my one and a half years old son is jumping up and down and writing on the table and wall. My three months old daughter is sleeping peacefully and all is well in my world.

I have been blessed with two healthy children, for which I did everything in my power to ensure they would be. I never wanted to look back and regret something I may or may not have done during my pregnancy.

I hope that you also will do everything you can to help your child's development within your body. You are its life source. Your every action must be done with the insight that you are carrying an innocent pure child. Everything you do, feel, and eat is going to affect your child.

I know this seems like an enormous burden to bear. It really is not. For just nine months you are the incubator to your child. It is such a short time within the span of an entire lifetime to be cautious of all that you do. If you are having a child it is because of a deep love that you have given to that little baby growing inside of you.

This is a time not only to nurture your baby, but also yourself. This is a time when you can reflect on past action and present and give yourself the time to have nothing but happiness and joy remain in your heart for these nine months. I know there are certain unforeseeable things that may occur while you are pregnant. You must try as hard as you can to be strong and not let anything deter you from your mission. A happy and healthy baby is what every woman wishes for.

You can have everything you wish for. You will take extra care of yourself these nine months. You will eat very well. You will rest as much as possible. You will smile always, and not only on the outside, but from within. An inner smile of joy is something very special. It is felt not only by your child, but also by your complete inner being.

This inner smile brings a certain tingle inside which releases chemicals into your system. These chemicals are what you wish to have flowing through you at all times during your pregnancy.

Although your child is not fully developed in the early stages of pregnancy, the embryo is still "aware". By this I mean that it senses everything that you are going through, physically and emotionally. I know that many women feel it does not matter what they do in the early stages of their pregnancy because it will not affect their child. Most women will not change their lifestyle until after their third trimester when they can actually see the growing of a belly and now know there is a child growing inside of them. Some women refuse to alter anything at all. This is so sad.

As soon as you have conceived everything you do will be a factor in the development of your child. The first three months are so vital to the health of your baby. Your child does its most growing and begins it neurological development in your first trimester. It is imperative that as soon as you find out you are pregnant you change your complete lifestyle to accommodate the baby growing inside of you. You will be thankful you did when your beautiful baby is placed in your arms.

My two children are both very happy and healthy babies. They rarely cry and slept through the night almost immediately after they were born. If they awoke hungry, it was a slight stir and a bottle soothed them back to sleep. I will say that I never woke my sleeping children to feed them. I don't care what anyone says; if your child is healthy it will wake when it is hungry. Never wake a sleeping baby to feed it if it is well.

My very happy babies are a joy not only to me, and my grouchy light sleeper husband, (he's going to have a fit when he reads this one!) but they are a constant delight to themselves. I know this may sound odd. A very happy baby whose demeanor is one of pure delight will advance and develop much quicker than children who are unhappy and cry a lot. This will happen to children whose mothers neglected themselves during their pregnancy.

Now almost a year later, my children are extremely happy and healthy children and are far more advanced than their age group. I am not saying I have child geniuses. I am saying that for their age they are socially more adept then others. By my children being so happy and healthy, they were able to devote more time to learning and socializing with others. They spent much time playing and laughing. I believe this is key to having a child acquire the skills needed to advance as a baby. They were mobile far faster than most other children. They were both walking by ten months. They spoke at a very early age, before one and a half year's old.

All children will eventually "catch up" with their peers very rapidly. Do not compare your child to others. Each child will develop at his or

83

her own pace. Your child is an individual, and will walk, read and write at his or her own pace. I am only saying that because my children were not crying they had more time to learn other skills and be more aware of themselves.

I completely believe that because they spent so much of their time laughing and enjoying being a baby, they were able to learn and absorb more. I know that the earliest stages of childhood do reflect hugely on their ability to achieve more during their life. Every day of your child's life is so important to its development into adulthood.

I know your child has just been born and already I have them in college and getting married, but it is very important that you do keep a constant focus on your child's happiness. A very happy and healthy baby is what you want and what I have been blessed with.

I completely believe that this is due to the fact that I stayed peaceful and happy during my pregnancy. I smiled a lot, and did not let little things bother me. I tried not to get angry at anything or anyone, especially my husband with all these hormones raging through my system.

My husband will tell you I was the woman from hell during my second pregnancy. Everything was his fault for nine months and I was only too happy to tell him. I made sure I found happiness in all aspects of my life. No matter what situation arose I came through it with a smile. Sometimes life brought me unexpected hurdles to face, but I always kept my inner smile glowing, and so will you.

Your brain is constantly releasing chemicals into your system based upon your moods. I completely believe there is good adrenaline and bad adrenaline surging through your body at all times. This release of endorphins runs also through your babies system. This is common sense and logic; what is in Mommy's system is in baby's system.

A happy Mommy means a happy baby to me. The more you can keep this happy flow of chemicals through your system and into your child's, the happier your child will be. Everything is a factor in your child's development.

A happy healthy you, means a happy healthy baby. Please don't have a major guilt trip if your child does cry a lot, or does not walk by ten months. All mothers praise their children and I am no exception. Though my children are adorable, happy, and healthy. My angels are far from perfect. If you did everything you could to ensure your child's health, all will be well. All children are unique, and your beautiful child will be happy with such a loving mom who cares as much as you do about his or her well-being.

Babies are individuals, but I believe you will increase your chance of having a very happy and healthy baby if you make every effort you possibly can.

CHAPTER ELEVEN

THE END IS JUST THE BEGINNING

Now is the end of my story and the beginning of yours. This is a time filled with joy, anxiety, laughter, and an inner strength that says you can do this. I have already completed my journey of giving life and it was wonderful. I would not have changed anything and am grateful that I can tell my children how great giving birth to them was, and how they helped me so much.

I would like to tell you a few things from my experience that may help you in knowing a little bit more of what to expect when you go into labor.

When my water broke, it happened instantly. There was no pain involved in this process. If you have ever stood up right after sex and had semen flow down your leg, this is what it feels like.

It is a thick watery discharge. It will continue to flow every time you move. Though they say the baby's head will act like a cork, water will

86

flow as you walk. This watery discharge will flow freely if your water happens to break while you are lying down.

If you are pregnant and are worried about your water breaking in public, you can buy "Depends" or use sanitary napkins to absorb the flow if your water does happen to break. I have heard people recommend using a panty liner. I personally would recommend a full size heavy flow sanitary napkin if you are worried about your water breaking in public or even at home.

I cleaned up quite a bit of water off of my mother-in-law's kitchen floor. I was lucky I was standing there when my water broke. I remember feeling so scared and using a lot of paper towels to clean up my mess. They were mad at me for cleaning the floor while I was going into labor, but I just couldn't leave this for her to come home to clean.

I was not wearing a sanitary napkin at the time of my water breaking. Most women's water will not break. Only a few percent of all pregnant women's water will break. Your doctor will most probably break your water after you have gone into labor.

To contain the flow of my water, I used a dishtowel, put big underwear on to keep it in place and held it between my legs till I got to the hospital. You can keep a towel with you also, just in case. You might just also want to be better prepared than I was, by wearing a sanitary napkin, in case your water does break. I was fortunate I was at home when it occurred, but it may have also very likely happened in public.

I know by the start of your third trimester, all you can do is think about the baby and all you have to do to get ready for its arrival. I hope this section will help prepare you a little bit more.

Have your bag packed at least two months before you're due date. Packing early will help to ensure you have everything you will need, and make sure no one will be going through your panty drawer finding items for you. Make a list of what you will need and check it off as you place the items into your bag.

I will tell you what I brought, also check other maternity books for help on what to bring.

1. Baby Blanket

2. Socks or booties

3. Onesies (if you think you may   be nervous pulling a Onesie over your newborn baby's head, buy snap t-shirts) Bring at least three.

4. Clothes appropriate for weather (A nice soft pajama, either light for summer or thick for winter, is ideal for baby)
* Do not bring anything in the bunting form. I found it hard to see where baby's legs   were when strapping my baby into the car seat.

5. Bibs (Bring at least three in case your baby likes to spit up, bring bibs with Velcro fasteners. Not snaps or string ties. You will find these difficult to use. It's easier to fasten the Velcro bibs around your newborns neck)

6. A small cap for baby's head (Make sure it is not too big, it may fall over baby's eyes or face)

7. Diapers (Newborn)

8. Baby wipes (I love Pamper's with Aloe) I found the gauze the hospital supplies is too rough for baby's bottom.

9. Balmex (I swear by this, my children never got diaper rash)

10. Burp Cloths, you will want to bring at least 6 with you just in case your baby spits up which will most likely happen. Be sure to put a nice soft cotton (terry cloth) burp cloth in your diaper bag to use after every diaper change to dry baby's bottom, before putting on a fresh diaper. This will help to eliminate diaper rash.

11. Desitin cornstarch powder with zinc (Do not use talc, there has been a risk of toxicity). If you have a boy never put powder directly on the opening of the penis (I read somewhere that some studies showed an increased risk of testicular cancer, this was with talcum powder, but why take any chances) Never put powder directly over your daughters vagina (risk of ovarian and uterine cancer), why take any risks with her too, (though it is harder for the powder to enter the vagina). I always sprinkled powder above my children's "privates", almost on their lower belly, and a little on their bottom over the Balmex, of course. *Another thing I always did after cleaning with a baby wipe was to pat dry my child completely. I never left any moisture on my child before I applied the Balmex or powder. My children never got diaper rash and I feel this was another reason why. I used burp cloths to do this with. Keep one in your diaper bag and on your changing table.

12. Car seat for infants (Give yourself plenty of time to adjust or readjust straps) Do not put hanging toys on your car seat. They are not approved by impact tests done in case you are in an accident. Always remember to put the handle of the car seat to the back when you are driving (Do not leave in up position, like when you are carrying the car seat) Have your car seat tested by a professional. There are many organizations that will test and make sure your car seat has been installed in your car correctly. If you have to buy two or even three car seats it is worth it for the safety of your child. Removing your child's car seat every time you change a car increases the risk that you may not have installed it correctly.

13. A book or magazine, Kindle, Nook, etc.

89

14. Camera or video camera (Don't forget the chargers, SD Card)

15. Large size plastic baggies and rubber bands (To secure any flowers you may have received). Put a little bit of water in baggie or wet paper towels and wrap around bottom stems of flowers. Place stems in baggie and secure with rubber band. It comes in so handy and you won't have to worry about water spilling in your car.

16. Cell phone, IPAD, laptop etc. and chargers

17. Address book for Thank You cards and baby announcements to send

18. IPOD (So you do not disturb others if you wish to listen to music at this time)

19. Some singles and/or a little bit of cash in case you want TV or food from the cafeteria

20. Bring any non-perishable snacks you may crave

21. Hair clips or scrunchies

22. Non-skid socks

23. Lip gloss or chap- stick

24. Slippers (You may get blood on them, so buy cheap, or a dark color, just in case)

25. Rubber waterproof shoes or "jellies" (When you use the shower you will want to go in with some protection on your feet. Showers are not cleaned after every use and there may be blood from other women who just gave birth)

26. Brush or comb

27. Extra contact lenses if you wear disposables (Bring case, saline, etc., if you don't)

28. Glasses

29. Two pairs of pajamas (Comfortable, cotton and V-neck (if you want to breastfeed) Not your favorite one, you may get blood on it.

30. Robe

31. Large size underwear, at least five or six pairs (In case you stain them) Make sure your underwear are cotton, roomy and comfortable. After you give birth you will be bleeding very heavily for a few days. You will have not only a large size medical bed pad folded up for protection, you will have TWO sanitary napkins on side by side too, stuck onto the medical pad. Don't worry the nurses will show you how to make it. You will be an expert mega sanitary napkin protector maker after the first try.

32. Comfortable, cotton bra

33. A couple of nursing pads, in case you start leaking

34. Very comfortable clothes and shoes to go home in (Keep in mind, the bulky sanitary napkins you will be wearing)

35. Toothbrush

36. Toothpaste

37. Soap (Some hospitals provide) carrying case or plastic bag to put in

38. Shampoo (Travel size)

39. Conditioner (Travel size)

40. Your razor, if you wish to shave

41. Washcloth and plastic bag to put it in when done (Most hospitals provide)

42. Eye cream

43. Face cream

44. Body lotion

45. Q-tips

46. Make-up

47. Deodorant

48. Blow dryer

49. Pen

50. The largest, widest, and thickest sanitary napkins you can find with wings (If you live near a wholesale store, buy a big box. You are going to need them)

51. If you have another young child, come prepared. Bring diapers for them, snacks and small toys they like.

52. You may also want to bring a breast-pump. Though it takes a few days for your milk to come in, if for any reason you have to stay

longer, you may need it. I have explained in greater detail on breast-feeding in Chapter 12. Check with the hospital of your choice, most hospitals will provide breast-pumps for you, if needed.

You may not need all of these items or you may even need more. Better to come prepared.

Going to the hospital will encapsulate every emotion you have. Make sure you are never more than a half –hour away from your hospital the last six weeks. You want plenty of time to make it to the hospital of your choice.

Have all your admitting forms filled out and pre-registered at the hospital. You will want your partner to be with you at all times by your side once you have gone into labor, and are now at the hospital. You will not want them filling out forms.

When you enter the hospital you will be brought to a birthing room. There you will take off all of your clothes, and place them in a bag the hospital should give you. They will give you a hospital gown to put on.

You will be asked if you can urinate so that they can check for dehydration (drink plenty of water throughout your pregnancy to prevent having false contractions due to hydration) and blood sugar level.

You will then be given a saline IV. to keep you hydrated and to have a place to administer medication if needed. There is no point trying not to get the IV. placed in you, trust me, I tried to refuse. If you are in a hospital they have to administer an IV. in case an emergency should arise.

You will then be strapped with a fetal monitor. This senses your contractions and keeps track of baby's heartbeat. A graph on paper with peaks noting your contractions and their intensity will continuously emerge from the fetal monitor machine. The nurses, doctor, and probably your excited partner will constantly check this. The baby's heartbeat will be on a screen on the machine. I personally never looked at this graph noting my contractions. I knew when they were coming and the intensity. I didn't need a piece of paper to tell me. My husband loved looking at it, though, and telling me a contraction was coming, and "wow" that was a big one, as the peaks flew off the paper.

Do not get excited if you are watching the fetal heartbeat monitor and the numbers rise and fall drastically, or even go off screen for a few seconds. This is normal. Each contraction will raise your child's heartbeat. If you happen to move the strap, the fetal monitor may not be able to pick up your baby's heartbeat, until you move again or the nurses readjust your strap. Please concentrate on your contractions and your child. Let the nurses and doctors check the fetal monitor. You do not need any added stress or worry. Your baby will do just fine inside of you anticipating its emergence into your arms.

You are now in labor, and there are a few different stages of labor that I will tell you about and what to expect. I will also tell you about the duration in most labors and I would like you to know that with your use of The Pod Method, you can confidently cut this time in half or even more.

FIRST STAGES OF LABOR:

LATENT- This stage is usually the longest, beginning days and weeks before without even the slightest notion from you, that it has even been occurring. Your cervix will begin dilating from one to three centimeters at this time. Your contractions if you even feel them will be relatively painless.

94

ACTIVE-   Your cervix will dilate from about three and a half centimeters to almost eight. It will usually take about an hour per each centimeter of dilation of your cervix.

This phase will seem like the longest because you will feel the most intense pain as your contractions intensify with every centimeter of dilation from your cervix. You will know your cervix is dilating by the frequency and intensity of your contractions. Your contractions will last almost a minute and will come every three and a half minutes. They will become extremely powerful.

TRANSITIONAL- This is the most important phase. The complete dilation of your cervix. This should not last long. Your cervix will complete its final dilation of ten centimeters. You will now feel the most intense pain as your child is now going to begin its descent once your cervix has fully dilated. Your contractions will be extremely frequent every two to three minutes at the most, and last about almost two minutes. You will feel the most pain of your labor now. But this phase is the shortest and helps to bring your beautiful baby into your arms. It will last on average from twenty minutes to an hour.

Once your contractions have begun, you will be checked and rechecked to see how far you cervix has dilated. Be prepared that more than one person may be sticking their fingers in side of you to do this.   They will check your cervix dilation in between your contractions.

Your water if not broken, will be done at this time. They use a long device, which actually looks like a knitting needle. It does not hurt at all. You will feel a warm fluid flowing out of you. The nurses will clean you right up and change the dressings on your bed.

Be prepared to have plenty of staff walking in and out of your room and all having a peek at your privates while your legs are spread. You will not care one bit, and neither do they. The only thing I remember thinking was, "Why can't they keep the door closed". I did not care about the nurses or doctors seeing me, just the people who may have been walking through the hall. Though after a few minutes even that thought completely went out of my mind, too.

You are going to be waiting for your doctor to say you can push now. This stage of labor can last from anywhere from 10 minutes to hours of pushing. This is the moment you have been waiting for. You have practiced pushing and will be able to help your child emerge swiftly.

Be prepared to have a nurse on either side of you grab a leg and either pull them out or push your legs all the way to your chest. I was not thrilled about this.

Once your baby's head is out, they will tell you to stop pushing so that they can suction out the mouth and nose of the baby. The doctor will also get a better grip on the baby to help it out. Sometimes the doctor will turn the baby slightly to help it emerge faster.

This may take a minute. It will seem like the longest minute you have ever experienced, with a baby half in and out of your vagina. It is not extremely painful, but it does not feel great either.

Once the baby is completely out there is no pain what so ever. All the pain is gone, wonderfully, magically gone.

There. That is it. You can and will do this. You are strong and powerful.

I know you think, that's it, it all over. You still have one more thing to do. Release your placenta.

As soon as your beautiful baby is out, focus on your placenta. Tell your placenta it did an amazing thing; you gave me a perfect little baby. Tell your placenta that it can go now, RELEASE, RELEASE. Concentrate intently upon your placenta to release. It will do as you wish.

I am telling you this, because if your placenta does not release, they may push forcefully down on your stomach or worse. Your doctor may have to put their hand inside of you and remove it. They will then manually scrape inside of your uterus with their hand to make sure the entire placenta has come out.

This thought has always made me wish if I were to have this done, that my doctor had very small hands. I have been told that this feels worse than childbirth. I believe anything that has to be done to you after the enormous stress upon yourself of giving birth will be compounded hugely in the pain factor. You are exhausted and sore; you will not want anyone even touching your vagina and birth canal at this time. I want you to relax and command your uterus to let go of your placenta. Concentrate and will your placenta to release.

When your placenta is ready to release; (this may take upwards of a half-hour), your doctor will push lightly on your stomach over your uterus and gently tug on the umbilical cord. There is no pain. Your placenta will feel oddly thickly gelatinous as it is expelled from your vagina.

I have never tried to see what my placenta looked like, and I would think you would have no desire too, either. Tell your partner not to look either. From what I have heard it is definitely not a pretty sight. Keep focused on your beautiful baby.

Start drinking water by the gallons, so to speak. Your IV will not be taken out until you urinate. Drink as much water as you possibly can, so that they will remove your IV from your hand or arm. I could not wait to get it out. I felt I did not need it in the first place, and it is extremely uncomfortable.

When you are ready to urinate, call a nurse so that she may help you to

97

the bathroom (you may still be a little shaky) and to show her that indeed you did go to the bathroom and you would like your IV taken out now (please).

You will experience soreness and some discomfort in your vagina and perineum area. It will hurt worse when you go to the bathroom. The more stitches you have the more it will burn at this time.

They will give you a squeeze bottle to cleanse this area with. Always make sure the water is warm. It feels great and helps to soothe and clean. The burning and soreness will get less and less every day, till it finally dissipates in a week.

Do not be fearful of having a bowel movement. Your stitches will not tear. Unless you tore all the way to your rectum, which is so rare, it is doubtful. You will not have any problem pushing out a bowel movement.

You will be monitored to see if you have had a bowel movement. Most hospitals will not release you till you do. If you have not yet had a bowel movement within twenty-four hours, tell your nurse or doctor. They will want to see if it is just nerves or another underlying cause.

It is so annoying to have any pain linger, no matter how small after you have given birth. I know I was not happy, and my discomfort was nothing compared to women who go through excessively long labors.

I felt I had just given birth, I did not want to endure even the slightest discomfort. I was tired, exhausted and just wanted to fully concentrate on my baby. But, the first week will fly by and be over quicker than you know. So will any residual pain.

Another event I was unprepared for was bleeding; this is called lochia. You will bleed heavily for almost two whole months. This is an inconvenience, especially if it is summertime. I thought I was going to bleed forever and having a sanitary napkin on twenty-four hours a day for two months was not enjoyable.

If you are bleeding very heavily (and by this, I mean so much blood it soaks right through your sanitary napkin) and with blood clots, you may be experiencing hemorrhaging of your uterus. Call your doctor immediately.

I bled heavily for two months. Every book I read said that the blood would taper off within a week and then I would experience light bleeding for a few more weeks. Every book stated I should have been completely done bleeding within six weeks.

I had a heavy flow for almost two months. Do not be alarmed if your blood flow does not taper off either. Do consult your physician just to be sure everything is healing right. Every woman experiences their bleeding differently. Some women may be done bleeding within a month, others longer. We are all individuals and our bodies will heal differently with each of us.

You can also not have sex until you have completely stopped bleeding. When you stop bleeding this signals that you are now healed and can now precede with sex and wearing tampons without the risk of infection. Your period will return within six weeks of giving birth, if you are bottle-feeding. Your period will return within 2-18 months later if you are breast-feeding.

Be also prepared that if you are going to breast-feed, you will have to wear a bra twenty-four hours a day with nursing pads, so you do not leak all over your clothes. This was something I had not even thought of when I decided to nurse. Finding a comfortable bra was the worse. Especially, for at night. I ended up wearing a very comfortable cotton sports bra with no under-wire.

You have no idea how hard it was to find a comfortable bra without under-wire. The under-wire would dig into my stomach, especially towards the end of my pregnancy. I found that a comfortable cotton bra helped me to sleep much better and had the extra comfort I needed.

It is not ideal for support, but I did not care. I wanted comfort. I went up to a 38D and my breasts have gone back to normal now. Buy several different bras. Keep comfort in mind for sleeping at night. Keep support for during the day.

Please do not be discouraged with all these minor inconveniences I am pointing out to you. I want you to be totally prepared for what will come. You have many choices to make. Awareness will help you to make the decision that is right for you. Look into your beautiful child's face and all inconveniences will dissipate.

I have stated some facts you should be aware of. Now, I would like to go back and give you in greater detail some facets of your labor. I will also tell you about C-sections and other different ways your doctor may have to deliver your child.

I will also tell you about breast-feeding. I implore every mother to breast-feed her child. I will delve deeper into the area of breast-feeding for which we as women have been blessed with this wonderful food source for our children, in the next few chapters.

CHAPTER TWELVE

NATURAL IS ONLY A WORD

Vaginal birth or C-section. Breast-fed or bottle-fed. There is no right or wrong, only the happiness of you and your child is what matters. Not the specifics, just the outcome, a very happy and healthy baby.

There are many ways to deliver your baby. I believe any way that your baby comes into this world is natural. Do not fret if you do not have a vaginal delivery. All that matters is your beautiful baby smiling upon yours. Natural is only a word and your baby emerging from your body is as it is supposed to be, naturally.

I know of many women who have felt they failed when they were told they must have a C-section. Why it is important to deliver vaginally is beyond me. As long as your baby is emerging from you, that is natural. Your child was not developed in a machine. That would be unnatural.

Your child grew within in you, as nature has made possible for the existence of our species. Anyway that your child must be delivered is of no consequence. It is the emergence of your child into this world and into your arms that is the miracle of life.

Never think you have failed in anyway, if your delivery is not as you had hoped. You conceived and helped to nourish your baby and that is not failure. That makes you a phenomenal woman in my book.

No one can ever know how there labor is going to proceed. There are numerous circumstances that may result in you having to have a C-section. A C-section is just another way out for your child. That is all, another way out.

Be thankful that our technology has advanced so greatly that we do have many alternatives for the successful delivery of our healthy, beautiful child. All that matters is our baby and that it gets out. When you are in your ninth month you will be thankful to have your baby out, no matter the nature of its delivery.

C-sections have successfully delivered more children than ever thought possible. This procedure has made for the significant decrease of death among our children emerging into this world. This procedure has saved so many children that most doctors will perform one if they feel there is the slightest risk to you or your child. Could you blame them? Why take any chances with the health of your child or yourself.

Do know that as with all surgeries there are always risks. It is now believed that though C-sections have helped deliver healthy babies in high- risk situations, they are also performed too much and too conveniently than need to be. This is still a major abdominal surgery. Never have this procedure performed because you think it is more convenient or you are scared of having a vaginal delivery. I have heard of some women requesting C-sections because they felt their vagina would stretch too much and they would not be able to please their partners after a vaginal birth! Can you believe this?

Vaginal is the best form of delivery of your child, but a C-section is needed if there is any complication during your labor. Some complications may be a breech baby, fetal distress, a prolonged labor with no sign of cervix dilation, and if your child's head or shoulders will not emerge through the birth canal. If you have any contagious disease of the genitals or a history of hypertension, kidney disease or diabetes a C-section will more than likely be performed.

There is a slightly higher rate of infant and maternal mortality associated with C-sections, then with vaginal birth. But if you need a C-section there is already a higher risk because of the fact you are even having this procedure done, due to complications. Do not worry; if you have a doctor you trust, you will know they have every capability of delivering your child safely into your arms.

With a major surgery of this kind, comes several factors, which you may or may not need. You may need a blood transfusion. This may come as a surprise to many women. But sometimes there may be an abundance of blood loss during this procedure if any complications arise. It is extremely rare nowadays for women to have a blood transfusion.

If you think you may fall under the category of having a high- risk pregnancy. You may want to talk to your doctor about storing your blood early on, if at all possible. You may even ask loved ones if they would donate and store blood for you, if the need arises. Discuss this option with your doctor. He will probably think me extremely ludicrous for even suggesting this, but I believe in trying to cover all bases.

You will also have to be prepared for the fact that you will need to stay in the hospital longer. Usually 5-7 days depending on the circumstances and your postpartum recovery. Make sure you have provided someone to watch your children for you, if this is not your first child. Even if you have successfully delivered naturally before, that is no guarantee you will deliver this way for each birth. Have a back-up plan ready so that if you do have a C-section; all you have to worry about is getting better and holding your newborn baby. You will not want to start calling everyone while you are on morphine from the pain to start worrying who will watch your children because now you will be in the hospital 3-5 days longer than expected.

If your doctor feels a C-section is necessary, have them explain to you all the situations why they feel you must have one. This will ensure that you know you have tried to deliver naturally, and that there is no other way for your child to emerge.

If there is immediate danger to you or your child, don't ask any questions. Get the baby out as quickly as possible. Ask questions after your child is sleeping peacefully in your arms.

Having a C-section is surgery. It will require anesthesia and painkillers after the birth of your child. You can now be fully awake during the performance of a C-section. You will be able to see your child as soon as it is born. Your partner or a loved one is also allowed to be at your side during the birth of your child.

You will be given an epidural. It is done by inserting a needle into your spine and administering painkillers constantly during the surgery. This will numb your lower body. You will be totally conscious of everything going on.

You will also have a catheter inserted to help you urinate. It will be removed within twenty-four hours of having your C-section.

104

More than ninety-five percent of all C-sections are performed by "Low cervical transverse" incisions. This is best known as the "Bikini Cut". You are given a horizontal incision right below the bikini line. This is a great relief to all women who will find that only they will know they have a scar from a C-section. Your pubic hair will cover it eventually. Plus the scar fades dramatically, too. You can still wear your bikini, mom.

You have had your epidural and now feel no pain. An incision will be made and your doctor will continue to cut through several layers of fat and muscle. Any internal organs like your intestines or bladder will be moved or even placed on your stomach. You will not feel any pain. You will feel your insides being moved around, this is an extremely odd sensation, and about the worse of this procedure.

When your doctor has reached your uterus a small incision will be made for your child to emerge through. Once your child is out your partner may still cut the umbilical cord if that is what you both desire. Let your doctor know before the procedure that you want to cut the cord. Most doctors will show you your child and ask if your partner wishes to cut the cord.

Your beautiful baby is here, and yes they will place your child next to you, if there have been no complications to your baby. You most probably will not be able to hold your child just yet. Don't worry; your baby will know it is you by your voice and your smell immediately. Stroke its cheek, and let your partner have these first few minutes to cuddle and bond with your child.

Now is the time to stitch you up. This takes the most time, usually a half-hour to an hour; depending on the skill of the doctor and bleeding you may be experiencing. Your doctor will clean out the placenta and clean out your uterus manually. They will then stitch up your uterus and make sure there is no bleeding left at all. Then your organs will be carefully put back into place. Then each layer of muscle and fat will

105

be meticulously stitched.

You will most probably get stitches or more commonly staples, to suture your main incision, which will be removed within a week. You will not be able to take a shower or bath until your stitches have been removed.

You will be drugged heavily with morphine. This will now be the worse time for you. You will feel drugged and nauseous. The total exhaustion and feeling sick will not be as worse as the pain of knowing you can't hold your child now even if they would let you, which they won't for several hours.

Relax. Get as much sleep as you can right now. You need all your strength. Your baby is more than likely sleeping peacefully in bed with a big smile on its face. Sleep, you have just had major surgery. Take advantage of this time to know that your baby is being well taken care of and you can sleep without any worry. Once you get home you will not have this luxury. Sleep.

The doctors will more than likely give you morphine as a pain- killer. They have also installed a pain relief dispenser, which you can administer to yourself as needed. This is so wonderful because you can dispense as much pain medication as you feel you need. Some women will not need as much as others. Each woman's pain tolerance level is different. Don't worry you can never overdose; there is a limit to how much medication you can dispense to yourself.

Depending on the circumstances of your C-section will determine when you will see your baby. Some women will want to hold their child immediately; others will want to rest and then see their baby when they feel they are a little stronger. There is no right or wrong. Do what you feel is right for you.

You will be asked to walk soon after the birth of your child. It will not be easy. But you must walk to ensure you are physically okay and to get the blood circulating again correctly through your system. You will only want to lie in bed after going through major surgery, but you will have to get up and walk. You will be asked to try to walk about ten hours to a day later depending on your recovery.

Most women will get up and go to their baby. This walk of love will help you to get out of that bed.

Be prepared to have sanitary napkins on at all times. Even though you did not have a vaginal delivery, you will still bleed. It will not be as heavy or last as long as if you had delivered naturally. You will begin to bleed within a day of your C-section, so be prepared.

Probably the worst part about postpartum recovery from a C-section is gas. I have been told that the gas can be so severe; it will debilitate you for a few minutes. This happens because when they open you up for the C-section, air enters your body and is then trapped when they stitch you up. This should only happen for about a week. Take a deep breath and sit or lie down immediately.

If you had planned to breast-feed, this is a difficult time for you. You will have to make a huge decision, right now. I know many lactation experts are not going to like my advice.

You have just had major surgery and have had anesthesia and pain-killers. These drugs do enter into your blood system and consequently into your milk supply. I highly advise that you do not breast feed your child until you are completely off of all pain relievers.

It has been medically documented that the drugs you are taking for pain do enter into your breast milk. The whole reason we as mothers are breast-feeding in the first place is because we want to give our child the richest and purest form of nourishment. Make your decision on the basis that there will be morphine and any other medications you had and still have to endure because of your C-section, in your breast milk.

I am a huge advocate of breast-feeding your child. I implore every mother to breast feed their child, even if it is just for the few days they are in the hospital. I know the first milk; the colostrum your child receives from you is the richest in antibodies and vitamins.

This is why I know you will have to make such a hard decision to refrain from breastfeeding during these first few vital days. I urge you to think about putting any known harmful chemical into your innocent child's system.

I highly advise you to pump your milk and then dispose of it. That is right; please throw it away. It is not pure. It is full of drugs. Do not give your innocent baby drugs especially since you are aware it is in your milk.

Your baby can drink formula to sustain it for the time it takes for the drugs to leave your system. This will be about forty-eight hours after you have completely refrained from any pain medication.

Do not let your child starve during this time. I don't care what anyone tells you, feed your baby. Lactation consultants are sometimes extremists when it comes to breast-feeding. This is your child; you must do what is right for you and your baby.

I and numerous other women have been told to not feed your child anything, until you have begun to lactate. This may take several days in most women. You will be told that your baby will be just fine if it is not fed for a few days awaiting your milk supply.

This is ludicrous, especially if your child was not heavy at birth. Your child will lose up to a pound after its birth. If you are not even feeding it, your child may even lose more. Remember, your child has to be at least five pounds for it to be able to go home.

If your child is crying, feed it. You may also be told that if you feed your baby with a bottle, you will then never be able to breast-feed. This is also not entirely true. Your baby is very smart. It will be able to go from bottle to breast without any problem.

This is also very handy to know. If you do breast-feed, you will then not be tied to your child twenty-four hours a day for however long you decide to breast-feed. You will be able to pump milk into a bottle and be able to leave your house to run errands or even get much needed sleep at night by allowing your partner to also help in late night feedings.

I know many partners who felt they were cheated by not being able to hold their child close and feed them a bottle while they rocked them to sleep. It will help immensely with the bonding of your child to others if they also have the opportunity to feed your baby.

Both of my children were breastfed for seven months. I used breast and bottle. I even used formula and breast milk. I was not blessed with an abundant supply of milk. I did the best I could. I started off every feeding with breast-milk and topped them off with formula if they were still hungry.

Now I hear the lactation community cringing and asking to have my books all burned. But, I really wish there had been someone who was there to tell me there is no right way. Each mother, baby, and situation is unique. There is more than one way to breast-feed your child and make sure it is fully nourished and satisfied.

I do not wish to offend the lactation experts in any way. I regard them as leaders of greatness and know that they completely hold your child's interest above any moral issues they may have personally. They know, as is also been medically proven that there is nothing on this earth that can substitute for nourishment as well as a mothers breast-milk. I am also an advocate of breast-feeding.

I only believe that they may not feel there are any other options available, only breast-milk. I just want to let you know if you are like me, and cannot sufficiently breast-feed your child that you can also bottle-feed and use formula to supplement your child's diet.

Please contact a lactation expert to help you with any questions you may have. They are more than willing to help with any area of breast-feeding you may need. They also have educational classes you can attend and experts are on call always. Contact your local La Leche League International Chapter. They are also affiliated with all hospitals and there will always be an expert available while you are at the hospital to help you get the suckling down right and answer all questions you may have.

As, I have always stated, there is no right or wrong. You must always go by your gut instinct and let that inner voice guide you to what is best for you and your baby. I just believe knowledge on every level is good.

I do urge you to breast-feed your child. I don't care if it is only while you are at the hospital, or until you return to work in six weeks. Better some than none at all. As I have said your baby will be able to go from bottle to breast without trouble.

If you really were not expecting to breast-feed, remember you can still bottle-feed also during this time, by pumping your breast-milk. I know most mothers do not want to breast-feed because of the time it consumes. But, by letting your child breast-feed, you will be giving your child antibodies and vital enzymes, proteins, and vitamins that will make a difference in the development of your growing baby. It will also make a significant difference for the health of your child with illnesses and making them stronger and healthier, which will last them a lifetime.

You can find it in you to breast feed for a few days to a few weeks, even if you were adamant on not breast-feeding. Remember everything you do from the time your child is born will reflect on its overall health in the years to come. Please breast-feed.

If for any reason you cannot breast-feed due to a medical condition or if you must take certain medications that are known to pass into a mother's milk, or even your child being lactose intolerant. Yes, if your baby is lactose intolerant even your breast-milk is harmful to your child. Do not be upset. All that really matters and the only thing that is the most important element to your child's happiness and well-being, is your love. I know that your love will be abundantly supplied.

I am not saying that you have to breast-feed for two years, though the women who have done this for their children should be sainted and given honors of recognition. It is such a dedicated and special mom who has the utmost patience and is totally unselfish who will breast-feed their child, especially for two years.

Breast-feeding is a special gift that we as women have been given to nourish our babies with. Why let this gift be wasted? I only breast-fed my children for seven months and that was because their teeth were rapidly coming in. If you wish to breast-feed longer please do, a lactation expert will help you to keep from getting nibbled and sore when your child's teeth start coming in.

A friend of mine who breast-fed for eighteen months told me she pulled her child sharply away when it bit her the first time and yelled, "No"! She felt awful when her baby started crying but she said it was a rare occasion that she was ever again accidentally bitten by her child.

Make sure your nipple and aureole is completely inside of your child's mouth. This will prevent soreness, cracking, and bleeding. I never

111

had any problems with soreness. I know a few women who stopped breast-feeding because it was just too painful and they were bleeding too much. Some women will definitely be more sensitive than others. Never feel guilty if you feel you have to stop breast-feeding your child for any reason. You are a wonderful mom for even trying and have given your child the most vital elements of your breast-milk from the first few weeks, or even days.

Another tip that helped me in keeping my breasts from becoming sore or cracked was something I recommend you to do, too. When taking a shower I never used soap to wash my breasts. I always just used water to cleanse naturally. Yes, shampoo and soap washed away down my breasts after washing my hair or face. But, I never scrubbed my breasts with soap or used a loofah or washcloth. I completely believe that since I left my breasts alone; I never irritated them externally by any chemicals. I never had any problems in seven months and hope you will consider this while bathing too. You may want to keep the water and bubbles or oils below your breast-line.

I also never put lotion on my breasts at this time. I creamed every other inch of my body except my breasts. First, I felt it may irritate my nipples and secondly, I thought my little baby would not be happy with the taste of my body lotion.

My children went from breast to bottle, bottle to breast without ever a pause. It was yummy food and they figured out real fast how to get the yummier of the two out, my breast-milk. I am telling you this so that you never have to worry that if you do not breast-feed immediately, you will never be able to.

I tried breastfeeding after my child was born. I honestly don't know how much breast-milk my child got in that first week till I really knew my milk had come in. I fed my baby a bottle as soon as I was given my baby at the hospital. I also sprinkled some milk onto my breast to let the baby suckle there too. This way he knew that there would

112

eventually be food here too.

My family all did not produce milk, though they tried. But, also back when I was born there was a lot less emphasis on breast-feeding. I knew I wanted to breast-feed my child, no matter how difficult it might be. Even in my best days whenever I pumped, the most I ever got out was one-and-a-half ounces of breast-milk, every 6 hours or so. That is why my children also got formula. I felt that as long as they got even a little bit of breast-milk during the day it was better than none at all.

I was glad that I was able to forgo drugs during my labor and therefore knew my milk was pure to breast-feed my baby with. I am sorry that you will have to make this difficult decision, but do know your baby is what comes first. I'm hoping you can relax and know that when your milk is pure again, your baby will not have any problem breast-feeding. Once he or she tastes that yummy, sweet milk they will have no problem suckling to get it out.

Again, please throw out your breast-milk and feed your baby with a bottle of formula. Formula is very pure and resembles a mother's milk so closely, your child will be provided all the nourishment it needs.

You will only have to forgo breast-feeding for a week at most. Less, depending on your level of pain tolerance. I know that in your breast-milk are essential antibodies that you will want your baby to acquire. Your baby will still be able to absorb these into their system once your milk is pure and free from chemicals.

If you are a die-hard breast-feeding advocate and cannot tolerate even the thought of formula going into your baby's system even for a few days. You may want to consider having your lactation consultant recommend a breast-milk donor. I have heard of breast-milk donors for women and for children in intensive care. They are usually nuns who have the utmost cleanest and purest milk you could find. Look into this option.

Another option is having a friend or family member who is breast-feeding at the time of your child's birth, pump some extra milk for your baby. Do this only with someone you completely trust and know. But these are just options. Most women should really not have a problem giving their child formula for a few days.

I only recommend that if you do give your child formula for a few days that you do not give them the formula with extra iron. I never gave my children this formula. Extra iron may cause constipation in newborn children whose system are not adequately used to absorbing food yet.

Also, I have read in numerous documentations that cancer actually feeds on iron in your system. Cancer patients are always asked not to supplement their diet with iron. I always felt that if there ever were the chance that there was any cancer present, it would have to starve and die. I would only allow the essentially needed iron for my children to develop healthy, and no more. I still do not use any food that says extra iron for my children and for myself. * *Consult expert on iron.*

My children, thank God, are both extremely healthy. Neither of them has ever had to have antibiotics, they are both rarely sick and each have never even had an ear infection.

Their stools from formula, was never constipated with the regular formula. Do not worry about your child being constipated with formula for the first few days. They should not have any problem absorbing the formula into their system. If you are worried about your child having an allergy to the formula, you may want to ask the doctor to recommend one for children with a chance of intolerance to formula. There are many formulas now for even the most sensitive baby.

114

You may want to use this formula for the few days it takes for your system and breast-milk to clear just to be on the safe side, if you have any reservations on using formula. Infant formula for highly sensitive allergic babies or who have intolerance for lactose; should be available at every hospital.

Most children though will not need this formula. If you are lactose intolerant or your spouse or any previous children, you will want to request this formula. If allergies run in you and your family, you may also want to request this formula too, just in case. Otherwise the regular formula will nourish baby just fine.

You will notice the difference between formula fed and breast-fed babies. Breast –fed babies stools smell like roses. Really! Since breast-milk is pure and sweet your baby's stools will be soft and sweet too. I sometimes couldn't even tell that my child had a bowel movement because there was never any odor. They always smelled like roses.

When I went completely to formula, there stools became a little harder and boy, you could tell when they had a bowel movement. You may find your child may be a little constipated going from breast-milk to formula. You may want to start slowly introducing formula to their system about two weeks before you completely abstain from breast-feeding them. It will also help their digestive system better assimilate to the difference in contents and help their bodies learn to absorb and digest formula better.

You may also want to do this if you have breast-fed your child till the age of one year's old. At one year's old you may give them milk. Whether you are using formula or breast-feeding, you will want to slowly introduce milk into their system also. Give your child the milk at the same temperature you gave them the formula, so that they will not reject it. Though it won't be long till your child will want their milk cold, straight from the fridge, usually when they are around eighteen months to two year's old.

If you are nursing your child it is extremely rare to conceive during this time. This is your body's way of protecting the milk supply for your baby; because once you are pregnant your milk supply will begin to diminish. Though the occurrence of conceiving while nursing is not likely to occur, it still can. If you do not want another child at this time or want to breast-feed your child for a set amount of time use a condom or practice very safe sex. You will not be able to use birth control pills until after you have finished nursing. If this was your safeguard against pregnancy before the birth of your child, consult your physician on another safe birth control method for now. Don't take any chances unless you want another child close in age to your fist born.

Now that you have all the knowledge to better make any decisions concerning you and your child on breast-feeding and what to expect from having had a C-section. I hope you will be able to decide what is best for you and your baby.

After a C-section you will not be able to sleep comfortably due to the cutting of your abdomen. It will be difficult to bend or lift the first few weeks. If you have a loved one who can stay with you the first week you are home from the hospital. You will be lucky you are so cared for.

Having someone to help with your baby will help you to rest and therefore get your strength back a lot sooner. If you cannot get help, rest whenever your baby does. Let little things go with house cleaning, if you can. Try not to do too much and just enjoy your baby.

There are two other alternatives to having a C-section. They are vacuum extraction and forceps. They are both used when your baby is not progressing down the birth canal or if your child's head is too large to fit through the birth canal.

These methods will only be used if you are in good health and there is no present danger to your child. Your doctor may take one of these options as opposed to forgoing an emergency C-section.

More than likely your doctor will use forceps to help your child emerge through the birth canal. These look like ice cube tongs, and are placed on either side of your child's head. Your child is then slowly and safely pulled out of your vagina.

The most likely risk with this procedure is the number of stitches you will endure by having forceps help your baby emerge into this world. You will require a longer cut and will more than likely tear or rip also.

Your child will be at a greater risk for head injury due to using forceps. But more than likely your physician would not even do this procedure if they even felt there was the slightest risk to your baby. Sometimes bruising and blood clots may appear on your child's scalp. These should go away within a few days. This is an extremely simple method of helping to delivering your child vaginally.

Vacuum extraction is used more abroad than in the United States. This method uses a cup adhered to your child's head, then held by suction. Your child is then extracted through the vagina. Though relatively safe the risks associated with this method are higher than with the use of forceps. You will more than likely not ever have this procedure done in the U.S. at this time.

CHAPTER THIRTEEN

BELIEVE

This book was designed to help you with all common phases of pregnancy. It may not cover every area and you should definitely consult other pregnancy books. I have given you powerful knowledge from my experiences and varied reading's from numerous books, the Internet, and what was told to me by expert OBGYN's. What I have told you is common standard knowledge involved during all aspects of pregnancy. I only wish to have stated it more matter-of-factly to give you a better knowledge of understanding to what will be occurring to you during your pregnancy.

I have hoped to give you supreme knowledge on this wonderful time in your life. Knowledge is power. Power is having a strong inner sense of who you are and what you know is best for you and your baby. Do not be swayed by me or anyone else in any area that concerns your child. Only you can make the ultimate final decision concerning you and your baby in any circumstances you both may encounter.

Giving life is the miracle that will fill you with more joy than you have ever experienced or even thought possible. Each pregnancy and baby is unique. No two pregnancies will be exactly alike. As, no two children will ever be exactly alike. This uniqueness is what makes us all individuals. What we can strive for is, all of our labors to be easy and for all of our children to be happy and healthy.

You have many choices and decisions facing you concerning your pregnancy and the birth of your child. The Pod Method is only to give you strength to achieve anything you set your mind to. Because it is used in the convenience of your home it makes it relatively easy to learn and use this method. It also does not conflict with any other childbirth methods. We urge you to seek out other childbirth methods and to use them in conjunction with The Pod Method.

There are so many choices you will have concerning the oncoming birth of your child. Using The Pod Method will be a relatively simple choice to make. But, you will have very difficult decisions that you will have to make with your partner. Will you home birth? Will you use a midwife? What position do you want to use during the delivery of your child?

I urge you to make a "Birth Plan". This entails down to the minutest detail your intentions and wishes on how you will want the birth of your child to proceed. I will tell you that if you have any medical conditions, a multiple birth, or have experienced any complications, and have had any previous problems with previous births, you will not be able to have exactly what you may have wished for. You will have to follow all of your doctor's advice and have your baby in a hospital.

If you do wish to stray from the normal routine delivery of your child, and by that I mean in a hospital with a doctor, I suggest you research completely your alternative method. You should also know that if you wish to not have your child in a hospital, you take a drastic chance with your life and that of your unborn child. It has been statistically proven that you increase the chance of risking harm to yourself and your baby by such a huge percentage that I highly recommend you take this into consideration when making your final decision. The risk of complication and death to you and your child doubles if you are not in a hospital.

Hospitals monitor you from the second you enter the hospital. Your doctor is fully capable of handling any situation that may occur. There is also a full medical staff available if needed. If any complication should develop, you are now with expert doctors and a full neonatal ward capable of taking care of your child for any occurrence that may arise.

You still may wish to have your child with the help of a midwife or "doula'" as they are sometimes referred to as. If you are not having any complications you can wish to be cared for by a midwife. You can also have your birth in a hospital with your midwife present to deliver your baby, with a doctor there or on call.
Midwives are trained in delivering your child and use methods, which many women have found to be of such comfort and help that they would never think of having a doctor deliver their baby. Midwives have at least 8 years of medical training and certification before they can be recognized as a Certified Nurse-Midwife (C.N.M.) by the American College of Nurse-Midwives. But they can still only deliver your child if your pregnancy and child have absolutely no complications.

I strongly recommend that if you feel you would prefer a midwife to a doctor; that you still have your baby delivered in a hospital. You will have the best of both worlds. A woman who will soothe and care for you and has now become not only your midwife but also a friend. You will have a doctor, a complete medical team, and a neonatal ward right there for you, if the need should arise.

I know many women are beginning to want home births. They feel the

120

medicinal and unfriendly atmosphere of a hospital is not how they want their baby to be delivered into. I will say to you that before you choose this option; take a tour of a few hospitals in your area. Hospitals have changed dramatically within the last few years.

Birthing rooms have been installed in almost every hospital. These rooms provide all the comforts of home. A nice big bed, that you will stay in for your entire labor and delivery. No more being moved from a labor room to a delivery room. A nice, big comfy couch, stereo and television are available. Most birthing rooms have their own private bathrooms for you to use. Hospitals have come a long way in making every possible accommodation for you to feel at comfort. I had a beautiful birthing room and every doctor, nurse and medical staff, were the utmost professional and extremely friendly. I loved every moment of my experience and would not have changed one thing.

I urge you to consider that in the event you are at your home and a complication should arise, the precious minutes it may take to get you and your baby to a hospital could mean the difference between life and death.

I know some women want their child delivered at home because of the fear of kidnapping. Please know that every hospital has state of the art security measures to ensure the safety of your child. I was given an electronic device band and so was my baby. If your baby goes within an inch of the obstetrical ward an alarm will sound.

Also, you can now have your child stay in your room until you depart the hospital. The only time your child will be taken to the nursery is when you request, or if your doctor has to check your baby, a nurse needs to give your baby a bath, and during visiting hours. This precaution is to protect your child from any germs visitors may be carrying, that may infect your child.

A major factor in the high rate of women wishing to have home births

121

is the increasing costs of having your baby in a hospital. My easy, short labor still cost about three thousand dollars. I was just so relieved to know that we were fully insured. The only bill we incurred that my husband was upset about was for the anesthesiologist. It was for six hundred dollars, of which we had to pay half. My husband and I both were incredulous when we got this bill because I never even met him. I never even took an aspirin my entire stay in the hospital. When we called to ask why we were being charged for a service we didn't use, we were told we had to pay for the anesthesiologist even if we didn't use him because he was "on call", just in case I needed him if an emergency arose.

So be aware that even if you have a drug free labor you will still pay the same cost as the woman who used drugs during her delivery. All in all, it was worth every penny to have our children born in a hospital. The peace of mind knowing that we were in the best place in case an emergency did arise during my labor; was well worth the exorbitant cost of a hospital stay. There isn't any amount of money to high to pay for the assurance of having a healthy smiling baby.

If you are planning for the birth of your child please make sure to have health insurance. Save some extra money if at all possible in the event a job is lost. Your employer will have to keep your health insurance going for at least twelve months. It's the law. This is called COBRA, you may want to check your company's policy and find out how much you will have to pay, in order to keep your health insurance active. You will have to pay a percentage of the cost of your health insurance. It is still much cheaper than finding a new provider with a baby already on the way. *DO NOT assume pregnancy is covered in your health plan. Check before planning to have a child each state is different Louisiana for instance makes you pay for a separate rider and takes months before it activates.

Please have everything in order and all premiums up to date. If for any reason you are caught off guard with an unexpected pregnancy and no insurance, you will still be given exceptional care with help from government assistance. But please be prepared with the upcoming birth of your child and your health insurance. This is very important to have in order and will give you one less thing to worry about. You never want to choose a home birth because it would be cheaper because you were not insured.

If you still wish to have a home birth, you may also want to think about all of the amniotic fluid, placenta, and blood involved in the process of birth. You will want your house to be clean and sterilized. You will be told, by your midwife; about what will be needed, like lots of clean sheets and towels.

I also recommend that you watch The Learning Channel's program, "A Baby Story". This show follows the births of women from their pregnancy, labor, and finally the delivery of their baby. Check your local station for airtimes.

Watching this show you will encounter many aspects of births that have been filmed for your viewing pleasure. You will see so many different "Birth Plans" that you will be able to see for yourself exactly what will happen to you if this is the method you also desire. I will be honest that I have watched some shows that strayed far from the norm of traditional childbirth, with my mouth hung open in complete amazement. You may reconsider a certain "Birth Plan" you had desired after witnessing another woman go through her experience. You may also reinforce your commitment to your "Birth Plan" after watching this show, also.

Along with your decision for the location you will want your child born, you may also want a certain position to be in when you deliver. I have witnessed on "A Baby Story" women giving birth standing up, squatting, doggie style, and giving birth in their bathtub.

I will say that these births have remained in complete remembrance in my mind. I was utterly stunned by these methods of giving birth. I will also have to say that I commend and admire these women for their strength in actually following through and sticking to their "Birth Plans".

It has been documented that standing upright or squatting has resulted in quicker labors and entails less of a chance of requiring an episiotomy or even the likelihood of tearing. The force of gravity pushing down upon you and your baby helps push your child out.

There really is no evidence of "doggie style", and by this I mean kneeling on all fours, to help or hinder the birth of your child one way or another. I will say that the woman I watched delivering this way, had all her family and friends present to witness the birth of her child. I was incredulous, because I could honestly say that I would never have my derriere naked in the air for all to see, no matter how "beautiful and natural" birth is supposed to be. I salute her.

Some women now want water births for their child. They feel emergence into this world from the amniotic sac into warm water will make it a less traumatic entry for their baby. There are many birthing centers that can accommodate a water birth. These birthing centers are usually fully capable of handling any medical emergency that may arise or are within minutes of a hospital.

The woman I saw giving birth in her own bathtub was completely naked and had her loved one seated behind her in the water with her. They had friends and family there to witness the birth of her child. I will honestly say that to be going through intense contractions while giving birth naked in a bathtub is completely not for me. I could not imagine that the severe pain you will experience during labor and then being confined to a porcelain bathtub, was a little extreme even for such an easy labor, as I had had.

Also the thought of sitting in a bathtub full of blood and fluids was something I could not even have imagined as a way of delivering my child. I could not imagine delegating the job of cleaning my bathtub after the birth of my child to a loved one. Please do not take offense if you have given birth this way, this is only my personal insight and thoughts to what I witnessed.

There are so many ways in giving birth to your child that I could not possibly name them all. Also every couple have their own little unique theories and methods of how they would like to deliver their child. All I ask is that you completely research any method that you may want to use for the birth of your child. Question, question, question; everyone and everything involved with your Birth Plan if it falls short of traditional. Please again think long and hard before you have your child outside of a hospital. You may end up with the easiest labor and regret that you did not have your child home as you had wished. But hindsight and wishing is good only if your outcome was a healthy mom and baby. Do not take the chance of regretting you were not in a hospital.

The Pod Method will help any Birth Plan you may choose in that having a fast, easy labor will put a lot less stress upon you and your baby. Less stress will probably result in less complication. If you are having a home birth we urge you to use The Pod Method as part of your Birth Plan. But, I still hope you change your mind and go to a hospital.

Also, some religious beliefs are based on the fact that the emergence of your child should be done with complete calm, tranquility and quiet. This is to lessen the trauma a baby encounters upon its birth into this world. They feel the child should not hear their mother screaming in pain, as they are coming down through the birth canal.

I always felt that The Pod Method would help these women immensely, to actually be able to forgo drugs and keep silent. Having a very easy, fast labor would not only help in making it an effortless delivery, the women would then be able to forgo drugs and have a less painful labor with use of The Pod Method. I personally commend these women for being able to go through an entire labor without uttering one word. Could you? This is really a labor of love.

Well I have tried to give you a broad range of subjects and methods to help you with your Birth Plan. Please remember that no matter what you had desired, may not always be able to happen just as you would like. Nature will proceed as it wishes and in its own time. Do not be disappointed if you had your heart set on having a home birth and could not, or wanted a vaginal birth and had a C-section. All of this does not really matter. You know what is more important than wishful outcomes of what you imagined your labor would be like these past few months. A happy and healthy baby to hold in your arms; is the only thing you should ever really desire. Everything else is inconsequential and just a prelude to the beginning of your life with your beautiful baby.

I have told you everything to help you on your journey of giving life. The Pod Method will help shorten your labor time and lessen the pain, by empowering you and dissipating all negative thoughts. If you truly believe you can have a quicker labor, you will.

The Pod Method is simple yet effective. By stressing the areas your pregnancy and labor will involve, you will be better prepared to handle any situation that will occur. The Pod Method was designed with one goal- to help you have an easier labor. Knowledge is power and you have been given an enormous gift of empowerment over your body to achieve this. Your gift; is a mind that has the power to obey anything you ask from it.

Your mind is an extremely evolved "machine" that is capable of performing amazing functions for you to adapt, teach, and use at will. This is the whole basis of The Pod Method, using your powerful mind to help you to achieve anything you wish. Whether it is a shorter labor

126

or accomplishing a dream, your mind is a tool you can hone to perfection.

You can have anything you desire, once you set your mind to believe it can be made possible. If you do not believe, it will never be yours. All your dreams and expectations will diminish along with your disbelief. If you do not truly believe you have been given an enormous gift; you will never be able to change your life or even help yourself to an easier labor. It all is intricately tied together. A deep belief in yourself will mean you can do anything you want. Everything is possible. Nothing is beyond your reach or control. You are the "Queen" of your kingdom. You rule over your mind, body, and house. It is yours to request, and it is yours to be obeyed. BELIEVE.

The mind is extremely powerful and you can do anything you wish. A shorter and less painful delivery will be yours if you so desire. Your mind and body will obey your demands and wishes. It is that simple.

Please remember that you are in control. It is your body. Never let anyone tell you that you are powerless in any situation that may occur to you in your life. The end of your labor is the beginning of your wonderful new life with a beautiful, happy, and healthy baby in your arms. BELIEVE.

CHAPTER FOURTEEN

A PERSONAL PLEA

Now that your beautiful baby is here you will want to maintain its health and development as best as you can. But, as we all know there are hidden dangers everywhere. In our food, our water, and even the air we breathe. It is a constant battle of knowledge to keep our children safe and secure. Knowledge is power. Awareness is vital for the continuing health of your baby.

Please check all ingredients on anything you may give your child. You just spent nine months ensuring the health of your baby. Remain always vigilant in this quest.

Some products I have come across; contain potentially harmful chemicals. These chemicals can be found in infant and children medication, teething pain medicine, toothpaste, and some foods.

One of these potentially dangerous chemicals is aspartame (phenylalanine, aspartic acid, and methanol are its three components; one of which methanol is a highly toxic poison). Aspartame is a chemical that should not be used in anything that will be ingested by a child or any pregnant mother- to- be. Nutra-Sweet is one brand that uses aspartame.

Saccharin is another potentially harmful chemical that may cause cancer if ingested. I have just heard recently on a news report that the FDA has taken saccharin off of its list of potentially hazardous chemicals. They have since stated that the link between laboratory mice and cancer was too small to make a connection. You have been given the knowledge; use this chemical cautiously as you wish.

I will add that my daughter developed an allergy to all artificial sweeteners. Her face gets puffy and swollen. She has horrible nightmares and screams in her sleep. It is very scary.
I know instantly if she has had this ingredient. There are many who get horrible migraines, rashes, swelling also and numerous other side effects. I pray to one day have these ingredients be listed very clearly on packaging as it is now slipped into bread, biscuits, gum, and other foods that really never used it till recently. The power of lobbying and I guess they think we are all obese in America and are doing us a favor. Little do they know how sick some are getting. Please call the manufacturer if you find any of these ingredients just listed. We should be made aware of anything artificial in our foods.

Maybe a new artificial symbol can be created that we can put on all packaging so even children would know what they might be ingesting. Fluoride is a deadly chemical that has been linked to cancer and Down's syndrome. Fluoride has also been recently introduced to our water supplies because this chemical has been highly regarded as a must have for healthy bones and teeth. Check your local water supply to see if this chemical is in your water. You can use filters to clean this toxin out of your water.

This poison is also in our toothpastes. There are toothpastes you can find which do not contain this chemical. You may want to use toothpaste made without fluoride until your child is old enough to have learned to spit out their toothpaste after they have finished brushing. Most young children will swallow their toothpaste until they learn it should be expelled.

This deadly chemical has now been combined with our children's vitamins. If your pediatrician wants to write you a prescription for vitamins with added fluoride, please request another formula, which does not contain this chemical. It seems to me completely unbelievable that they would put this chemical into our children's vitamins.

There are many children's vitamins on the market, which do not contain this or any other potentially harmful chemicals.

These chemicals are regarded as safe in low quantities of ingesting. The potentially scary and unsafe use of these chemicals is that they are shown "Not to be disposed of " by our bodies; but rather our bodies accumulate these toxins over the years. This is where the potential hazards exist.

Remember to check all your ingredients on anything you and your children will be using. It is amazing that we would have to even worry about toothpaste. But danger is everywhere, and we must always be alert of new chemicals and old ones that are being introduced into our systems.

You will also have to vaccinate your child. I believe that since it is law that we have our children vaccinated, to stick with the tried and true basics. I have refused every new vaccine, which has come into the market over the past few years. Please be educated on the risks associated with new vaccines. Their potential for harm to your child will be higher.

A recent vaccine, which was introduced to the market I refused to give my children. My doctor asked me at each visit if I was sure I did not want it for my children. I refused. It is not your doctor's fault; they are believers of helping and preventing illnesses to your children. These vaccines are supposed to prevent illness not cause it. Well, I now am so glad that I did refuse this new vaccine. It was pulled off the market after a year due to it causing children to get very sick and horribly some were killed because of this new vaccine.

If you feel strongly about the great benefits of vaccinations, please use extreme caution on giving your child a newly developed vaccine. I would urge you to wait at least a year after its arrival onto the market, before you give this new vaccine to your child. Unless your child has a health risk and you feel strongly that the vaccine will protect your child and the benefits outweigh the risks, you will do as you wish. It is your child and only you can make this decision.

Please stick to the basic vaccines, mainly because we have to, or we cannot even put our children in school. There are many organizations and groups who are trying to stop the mandatory inoculations of our children. They believe these vaccines are not needed and cause many diseases, including cancer. They feel the side-effects, risk of acquiring the disease you are trying to prevent, and death are just too extreme to take a chance with our children. There are some who have home schooled their children so they would not have to vaccinate their children.

I knew I needed the basic vaccines and since home schooling was not an option though I wish my family and the culture we live in was a lot more tolerant of this method of education. Because of my fear of vaccines due to all these substantiated reports, I also never got flu shots for my children. Why introduce any foreign antibody into their system, unless it was absolutely necessary.

My children are very healthy and maybe I do have the luxury to pick and choose as I wish. If your child has any medical conditions that a vaccine may help them to prevent a life-threatening disease you must listen to your doctor's advice. But, please be fully informed on everything, including side effects involving any new drug or chemical you will be giving your child.

Please know that if you are a devout vegetarian each time you have a vaccine you are inserting animal into your body. Read the ingredient list of most vaccines which contain monkey or bovine and other animal products. Join the club, I just found out myself......

Another area of well-being for your child is the well-being for you and others who will take care of your child. This is such a new experience. There will be days when everything is great and wonderful and there will be days filled with stress. This is life.

No matter how wonderful a mom you are, sometimes your child will cry, and there will be nothing you can do to stop his or her emotions from finally coming to a conclusion. Yes, even my perfect angels have cried and cried and cried. One phrase, which I have always remembered and has gotten me through the tough times of a child crying is, "No child has ever died from crying". This simple phrase has helped me enormously when I have tried everything to soothe my child and begin to scare that something is extremely wrong.

This phrase has been also taught in anger-management classes to control a person's temper that may be directed at a crying child.

It is recommended that if you do have a violent temper to remember this phrase, put the child down safely in bed and close the door slightly and leave the room. Wait until you have calmed down before you approach the baby again or call someone for help. Most times, the baby will cry themselves gently to sleep.

Be aware of anyone who will be staying with your child, even a loved one. Never jeopardize the health of your child. I have heard of horrible stories where a trusted person had a violent temper and shook the baby and caused its mental retardation. This is a personal plea of mine, be aware. Your child is counting on you to protect it from harm.

Always use your gut instinct when it comes to you and your child.

When my child is crying when I am driving (never take your child out of the car seat), or if I am taking care of my other child, or just trying to go to the bathroom, I always remember this phrase.

If your child will not stop crying, take a deep breath and sing a happy tune, knowing that they will eventually stop or fall asleep. Think of it as exercising their lungs. Never shake a child or hit them. Check for fever, soiled diaper, hunger, something pinching on their skin, teething, pulling on their earlobes (could be a sign of an ear infection), use your maternal instincts. If their cry is a fierce cry and a sound that really scares you, call your pediatrician or take them immediately to the emergency room.

Most children cannot relate what they want or what they are feeling in words, so they know crying will get your attention and will help them get what they desire. Sometimes all they want is to know your there and they will be soothed eventually in your loving arms.

Another thing that I always did was never to leave my children out of my sight. I never even bought a child monitor. These devices are meant to allow you to be away from your child for hours at a time and give you a feeling of safety. Now they even have video cameras to monitor your child with. I believe that no device can ever substitute for a mother.

I received a bassinette or "Moses bed" as they are sometimes referred to as by my Aunt Zory who made it by hand for me. My children both slept in this bed from the day they came home until they could no longer fit in it.

Since I could carry the bassinette with me everywhere I went, I always could watch my children myself. I took my sleeping child with me from room to room and always had them in view. I found this bed invaluable to have and highly recommend you put one on your baby registry. This bassinette is also great to have when you visit loved ones or are sleeping away from home. Your baby always has a nice soft, familiar, and comfortable bed to sleep in.

With the fear of SIDS (Sudden Infant Death Syndrome), I knew nothing could replace a mother watching over their baby, themselves. I even kept my child by my side as I slept. Maybe I do take things to extreme, but I always feel better safe than sorry. I would never take any chance with my baby.

I know there was one time when my baby was sleeping on his back; as is now recommended by doctors to prevent SIDS. My baby threw up his food so forcefully it flew out of his mouth and came right back into his mouth and down his throat with such force, that he immediately started choking. I thank the angel's every day that I was there. He was only one month old and if I had not been there to immediately turn him over and help him to expel, I don't even want to think of what might have happened.

Please never feel a sense of false security with any device. Never leave your child out of sight. It is said that your child's chances of SIDS decrease after three months and fall to a very low percentage rate by six months. I know my mother and mother-in-law; both breathed a sigh of relief as each of their grandchildren turned six months old.

I know that a child monitor does come in handy and there were times when I wished I had one. If you do have a child monitor, just please keep in mind that it does not replace you. Keep a constant watch over your child always.

You may also want to never turn down your radio or TV while your baby is sleeping. Putting a "ssshh, baby's sleeping" sign on your baby's room and tiptoeing around the house will surely make your life intolerable. By this I mean, if you train your child to only sleep when it is very quiet, you will end up with a very cranky, crying baby on your hands.

Most moms begin this system of putting their child to sleep, because they are usually home alone with them during the day. This system is fine, but you can't always guarantee your baby peace and quiet while it is sleeping.

I never changed anything going on in my house or surroundings to accommodate my sleeping children. This has turned into a blessing and helps to make my life and others so easy, as to not have to constantly worry that everything you say or any noise you make will result in your baby waking up.

I now have two children who will sleep soundly and peacefully, through anything or any noise. They will not wake up if I drop a pan, or am watching TV, and if company is over they can talk laugh and have a great time without worry. This is so great to have instilled in your baby, because you will probably have more children and it will be much harder to enforce a "quiet rule" with your new baby and a rambunctious older toddler sibling running around.

My husband is huge Nascar fan and has to watch the car races with the volume turned way up on the television, to get the "full effect" as he calls it. During the races, which last several hours, it was so great to be able to leave my child nearby, sleeping soundly in the bassinette. My husband could watch the baby and his race, just the way he likes to, without waking our sleeping angel. I was able to get some chores done without worry. My children both love "race cars!" now. I find this so wonderful; because my husband can now turn off their favorite cartoon and they will not complain once they see the race- cars roaring around the race- track.

Raising my children to not wake at the slightest noise has made my life and theirs one of joy and ease. I can now continue my day without my life coming to a standstill every time my child takes a nap. I can also take my children in and out of the car without waking them. I can also dress them or even change their diapers while they are sleeping soundly. Please take this all into consideration when giving your baby a nap. It will make a huge difference in the months ahead and will make your life one of ease, also. You will have a very happy well-rested baby to enjoy.

Please do not be offended by anything in my personal plea. I know that you as a loving mother already know exactly what needs to be done for your child and you don't need me speaking my mind. But all of these things I have mentioned have helped me, and it can't hurt to mention them to anyone else with a child. We can never know or be educated too much when it comes to the safety and health of our children. We have devoted every waking moment since the day our baby was conceived to give them a beautiful and happy existence filled with our love. This constant awareness for our children will follow them throughout their lives and our own.

We have come a long way in our journey of giving life. We have exhilarating memories that we can share with our children, as they grow older. We have done everything we could as moms to prepare ourselves, and our children to face the world with strength and vitality. We have succeeded in creating life with a beautiful baby that has given us all a new meaning for the word "love". And I say to you, as you are rocking your beautiful baby in your arms, smiling down upon them as you close my book, "Congratulations to you, Mom".

BELIEVE.

APPENDIX A

THE POD METHOD VISUALIZATION TOOL
(located in back of your guide book)

Fill in your due date where specified
Place in a picture frame or tape to wall
Place The PMVT in a location where you will spend most of your time, and will be able to visually concentrate on it

VISUALIZATION STEPS (Refer to Chapter Eight)
Envision that the black circle is your cervix
The yellow circle is your child's head emerging from your cervix
Count form 1-10, commanding your cervix to open rapidly
Tell your child to get out quickly, help Mommy and GET OUT
Think words like cavernous, big, roomy, and large as you stare at the black circle (your cervix)
Command your cervix to OPEN, OPEN, 1 to 10 AS FAST AS YOU CAN, OPEN
Envision your due date, (always thinking a week before is okay). This is when you will want your cervix to obey your commands and open rapidly
Mentally and visually concentrate on The PMVT daily, and as often as you can during your day

APPENDIX B

BRIEF SUMMARY OF THE POD METHOD STEPS

1. BELIEVE

2. Visualize your due date

3. Banish all doubt from your mind

4. Command your body to know that it will have an easy delivery

5. Talk often to your child

 6. Tell your child to grow healthy and strong

7. Teach your child how to help Mommy

8. Tell your child when the time is right (your due date) GET OUT

9. Tell your child to keep its head down

10.Tell your child you love them, and cannot wait to hold them in your arms

11.Never say you love being pregnant, say you cannot wit to hold your child in your arms

12.Mentally and visually command your cervix to open rapidly

13.Use The PMVT and all of your Pod Method steps everyday

14.Do not exercise

15.Do not do Kegel's

16.Have lots and lots of sex with a 360-degree motion (consult physician)

17.Practice finding the right muscles to push with

18.Command your body not to feel the pain

19.Teach your mind and body that it will make the pain, "GO AWAY"

138

20.Take a multi-vitamin and extra folic acid (consult physician)

21.Stay calm and happy

22.Mentally and visually use The PMVT everyday

23.Repeat: I will do this. I control my body. No one can tell me I can't have whatever I want and I want a fast, easy, and less painful labor for the birth of my baby

24.Be aware

25.Always remember, "Knowledge is power"

26. BELIEVE

APPENDIX C

RECOMMENDED READING & USEFUL INFORMATION

What To Expect When You're Expecting
Arlene Eisenberg, Heidi E. Murkoff, Sandee E. Hathaway
Workman Publishing, New York

What To Eat When You're Expecting
Arlene Eisenberg, Heidi E. Murkoff, Sandee E. Hathaway
Workman Publishing, New York

The Pregnancy Book For Today's Woman
Howard I. Shapiro
Harper Perennial

The Girlfriends Guide To Pregnancy
Vicki Iovine
Pocket Books

Prescription For Nutritional Healing
James F. Balch, M.D., Phyllis A. Balch, C.N.C
Avery Publishing Group
.

LA LECHE LEAGUE INTERNATIONAL- 1-800-LA-LECHE

AUTO SAFETY HOTLINE- 1-888-DASH-2-DOT (To check the correct installation of your infant or child seat) or contact:
THE NATIONAL SAFETY COUNCIL-
http//www.nsc.org/airbag.htm

AMERICAN COLLEGE OF NURSE-MIDWIVES- (202) 289-0171
(To check for a midwives credentials)

THE LEARNING CHANNEL- www.tlc.com

CENTER FOR DISEASE CONTROL: www.cdc.gov.

****Please note that I am recommending these books based on my varied readings during my pregnancies. They do not constitute an endorsement from the authors listed.

****St. Ives Collagen and Elastin and Nivea Lotion do not promote their products to eliminate stretch marks.

APPENDIX D

BIBLIOGRAPHY

What To Expect When You're Expecting
Arlene Eisenberg, Heidi E. Murkoff, Sandee E. Hathaway
Workman Publishing, New York

The Pregnancy Book For Today's Woman
Howard I. Shapiro
Harper Perennial

Prescription For Nutritional Healing
James F. Balch, M.D., Phyllis A. Balch, C.N.C
Avery Publishing Group

I wish to thank these authors in particular for keeping my book as factual as possible. I hope I do you justice and kept up to the high standards you maintain. I would also like to thank the Doctors and OBGYN's through the years who have given me such valuable and detailed information on pregnancy and childbirth.

APPENDIX E

QUESTIONNAIRE

1. Did you   a) Buy this book?   B) Receive as a gift?   _____
2. How old are you?   _____
3. Is this your first child?   _____
4. If not, how many children do you have?   _____
5. How long was each labor? 1st_____2nd_____3rd_____
   If more than three please fill in_____
6. When did you start using The Pod Method?   _____
   _____

7. Did you feel The Pod Method helped you to have an easier labor?
   _____

8. How long was your labor using The Pod Method?   _____
   _____

9. Will you use The Pod Method again?   _____
   _____

10. Will you recommend The Belly Bible?_____
   _____

11. Comments: _____

   _____
   _____
   _____
   _____
   _____

Please mail to:
The Belly Bible
PO Box 266
Holtsville, NY 11742

*Send address for a free gift as Thanks from us!
Name:_____

Address:_____

City, State:_____

Zip Code:_____

INDEX

A

148

149

L

Labor-
      Latent- 115
      Active- 116
      Transitional- 116

Lactose Intolerant- 137, 142

Lamaze- 23

Lanugo- 28

Laxatives- 39

Leg Cramps- 50

Lidocaine- 94

Listeria- 42

Lochia- 121

Low Cervical Transverse Incisions- 129

M

Maternal-Serum-Alpha-Fetoprotein-Screening- 33

Meconium- 28

Medicine- 38

Metal detector- 42

Microwave Oven- 42

Morphine- 130, 131

Multi- Vitamin- 41

N

NAOT Shoes- 51

Nausea- 25, 41, 92

Nesacaine- 94

Neural tube Defects- 33

Nivea Lotion- 50

Novocain- 31

Nutra-Sweet- 36, 160

O

Oxytocin- 80, 95-96

P

Pain Control- 76

Pap Test- 27

Perineum- 54, 120

Period- 121-122

Phenylalanine- 37

Pitocin- 95

Placenta- 46
        Manual extraction- 118
        Previa- 51, 80
        Releasing- 118

PMVT – 71-74, 171

Preeclampsia- 53

Psoriasis Medication- 35

Q

NOTES

NOTES

NOTES

NOTES

MY BIRTH PLAN

DUE DATE –

OBSTETRICIAN- Name
                Phone number-
                Recommendations-

MIDWIFE/DOULA- Name-
                Phone number-
                Recommendations

CHILDBIRTH METHOD-

CHILDBIRTH CLASS-
                Time-
                Dates-

CHILDBIRTH COACH-

WHERE? Hospital- Addresss-
                Phone number-
         Birthing Center- Address-
                Phone number-
      Home-
      Other-

HOW DO YOU ENVISION THE BIRTH OF YOUR CHILD?

_____

_____

_____

_____

_____

_____

_____

_____

_____

DRUGS-None-
      Yes-

EPISIOTOMY-

POSITION IN   LABOR-

LOVED ONES PRESENT FOR BIRTH OF YOUR CHILD-
No-
Yes- list-

LOVED ONE TO HELP BRING BABY INTO WORLD- No-
 (you must have advance permission)   Yes-

CUTTING OF UMBILICAL CORD- Doctor-
                       Loved one-

BREASTFEED-No-
        Yes-

VIDEOTAPE EVENT-No-
           Yes-

NOTES-

_____
_____
_____
_____
_____
_____
_____
_____
_____
_____
_____
_____
_____
_____

IMPORTANT PHONE NUMBERS-

_____
_____
_____
_____
_____
_____

About The Author

Two angels make for a deliriously busy, full of surprises, and happy home. Married fifteen years to the most gorgeous man, "Lust and Love at first sight" has kept us committed to see our golden years meld into glistening sunsets shared reminiscing the memories that make family…..

May you share those special moments where words are not spoken but yet heard by your hearts with loved ones who adore you.

www.ingramcontent.com/pod-product-compliance
Lightning Source LLC
Chambersburg PA
CBHW060310290526
45789CB00001B/474